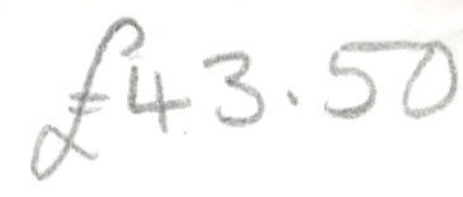

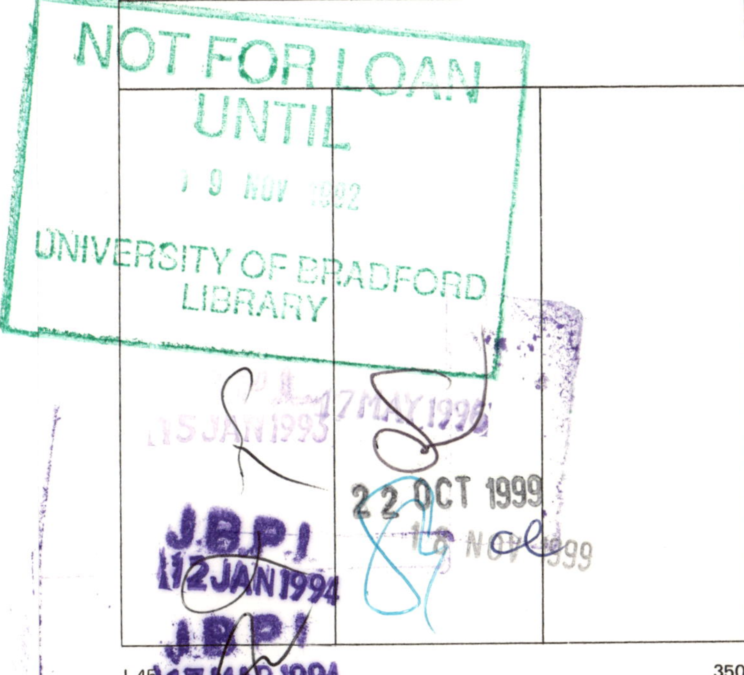

Immunotherapy and Vaccines

edited by
Stanley J. Cryz

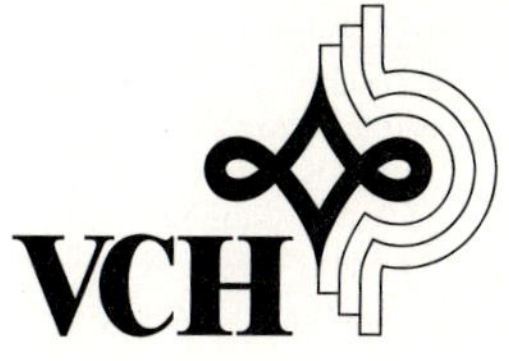

Distribution:
VCH, P.O. Box 101161, D-6940 Weinheim (Federal Republic of Germany)
Switzerland: VCH, P.O. Box, CH-4020 Basel (Switzerland)
United Kingdom and Ireland: VCH (UK) Ltd., 8 Wellington Court, Cambridge CB1 1HZ (England)
USA and Canada: VCH, Suite 909, 220 East 23rd Street, New York, NY 10010–4606 (USA)

ISBN 3-527-28098-7 (VCH, Weinheim) ISBN 0-89573-969-0 (VCH, New York)

Immunotherapy and Vaccines

Edited by Stanley J. Cryz

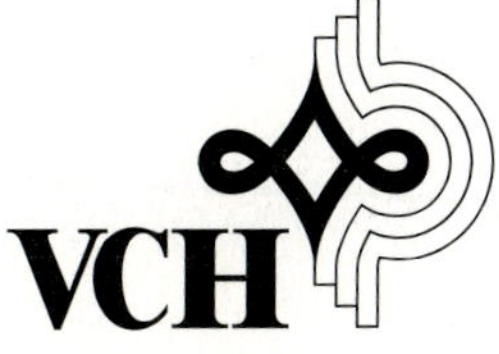

Weinheim · New York · Basel · Cambridge

Dr. Stanley J. Cryz, Jr.
Director Research and Production
Swiss Serum and Vaccine Institute Berne
P.O. Box 2707
CH-3001 Berne
Switzerland

Published jointly by
VCH Verlagsgesellschaft mbH, Weinheim (Federal Republic of Germany)
VCH Publishers, Inc., New York, NY (USA)

Editorial Director: Dr. Hans-Joachim Kraus
Production Manager: Myriam Nothacker

Cover illustration: TWI, Gestaltungsgruppe für Technisch-Wissenschaftliche Information
D-6943 Birkenau

A CIP catalogue record for this book is available from the British Library

LOC Card No. applied for

Deutsche Bibliothek Cataloguing-in-Publication Data:
Immunotherapy and vaccines / ed. by Stanley J. Cryz. – Weinheim ; New York ; Basel ; Cambridge : VCH, 1990
ISBN 3-527-28098-7 (Weinheim . . .) Gb.
ISBN 0-89573-969-0 (New York) Gb.
NE: Cryz, Stanley J. [Hrsg.]

Printed on acid-free paper.

Composition: Kühn & Weyh, D-7800 Freiburg. Printing: betz-druck gmbh, D-6100 Darmstadt 12. Bookbinding: J. Schäffer GmbH, D-6718 Grünstadt.
Printed in the Federal Republic of Germany

Preface

To control infectious disease, the medical community relies upon three approaches of prevention: (i) active or passive immunization; (ii) disruption of transmission via improvements in sanitation and nutrition; and (iii) treatment with antimicrobial agents. Each has had its share of successes and failures. Given the current socioeconomic status of the world, one can not reasonably expect a marked improvement in the living standard seen in developing areas in the near future. Treatment of infectious diseases in such regions is hampered by the comparative high cost of medical care and a lack of health care infrastructure. It would, therefore, appear that our reliance upon immunization as the primary means to control infectious diseases will increase.

The same conclusion also applies to developed areas of the world. Although in absolute numbers, the burden due to infectious disease is small compared to underdeveloped areas, new challenges continue to be presented. Advances in our ability to care for critically ill patients, increasingly complicated surgical procedures, and the expanded use of immunosuppressive therapy in treatment of cancer has led to a dramatic rise in hospital-associated infections. In many instances, antibiotics are of only modest help, in large part due to the freuency of resistant strains. New infectious agents, such as the Human Immunodeficiency Viruses, will undoubtedly continue to challenge us (even more so in underdeveloped regions).

Mass immunization campaigns at national levels have had a dramatic impact upon certain diseases, especially those where man is the only host. The eradication of smallpox is the best example. With the vaccines available for use today, we have the potential to also eradicate measles, mumps, rubella, polio, diphtheria, tetanus, and perhaps, pertussis. However, unexpected problems can arise. The number of measles cases in the United States has risen dramatically in the past 2-3 years even in the face of vaccine coverage which ranges from 92-97%. This is the result of a combination of two factors: (i) disease among children who either did not receive vaccine or did not respond to vaccination; and (ii) a drop in titer to nonprotective levels. A two-dose-immunization schedule has recently been recommended. Surprisingly, a large percentage of the adult population in Europe and North America has been found to be nonimmune against diphtheria and tetanus due to nonadherence to recommended regular boostering with these vaccines.

Hopefully, the present work will illustrate the point that the fields of vaccines and immunotherapy are far from static. Technological advances in molecular genetics, biochemistry, and cell biology have led to a burst of activity within the past decade. Never have more vaccines of such varied types been under study than as at present. IMMUNOTHERAPY AND VACCINES will provide a concise overview of the field concerning vaccines currently in use and those under development. It should, therefore, serve as a reference for workers in the fields of primary health care delivery, public health, and applied and basic research.

Berne, September 1990

Stanley J. Cryz, Jr.

Abbreviations

AIDS	acquired immune deficiency syndrome
BCG	Bacillus Calmette-Guérin
CMV	Cytomegalovirus
CPS	capsular polysaccharide
CS	circumsporozoite
Da	dalton
DNA	deoxyribonucleic acid
DPT	diphtheria-pertussis-tetanus
DPT-Pol.	diphtheria-pertussis-tetanus-polio
DT	diphtheria-tetanus
FHA	filamentous hemagglutinin
HBIG	human anti-HBV immune globulin
HBsAg	hepatitis B surface antigen
HBV	hepatitis B virus
HIV	human immunodeficiency virus
HRIG	human rabies immune globulin
humab	human monoclonal antibodies
Ig	immunoglobulin
IPV	inactivated polio vaccine
ISG	immune serum globulin
ITP	idiopathic thrombocytopenic purpura
IU	international units
IVIG	intravenous immune globulin
Lf	limit of flocculation
LPS	lipopolysaccharide
MMR	measles-mumps-rubella
NANP	asparagine-alanine-asparagine-proline
NVDP	asparagine-valine-aspartic acid-proline
OPV	oral polio vaccine
PFU	plaque forming units
PT	pertussis toxin
RESA	ring-infected erythrocyte surface antigen
RNA	ribonucleic acid
TCID	tissue culture infectious dose

Authors

STANLEY J. CRYZ, Jr., Swiss Serum and Vaccine Institute Berne, Switzerland (Chaps. 1 and 2)

MARTA GRANSTRÖM, Departments of Clinical Microbiology and of Vaccine Production, National Bacteriological Laboratory, Karolinska Hospital, Stockholm, Sweden (Chap. 3)

BRUNO GOTTSTEIN, Institut für Parasitologie, Universität Zürich, Zürich, Switzerland (Section 4.1)

LUC PERRIN, Division d'Hématologie, Hôpital Cantonal Universitaire, Genève, Switzerland (Section 4.2)

ALAN CROSS, Department of Bacterial Diseases, Walter Reed Army Institute of Research, Washington D.C. 20307-5100, United States (Chap. 5)

JAMES LARRICK, Genelabs Incorporated, Redwood City, California B40C3, United States (Chap. 6)

Table of Contents

1. Introduction

S. J. Cryz, Jr.

1.1 Historical Aspects

Immunization is the most efficient, cost-effective means of preventing infectious diseases. The concept of preventing disease by vaccination is an ancient one: in China and India, the practice of "variolation", whereby small quantities of material from disease pustules were used to immunize people against smallpox, was practiced before 1 000 B. C. The first "rational" approach to vaccination was taken by Jenner in 1798, who used naturally attenuated cowpox to immunize against smallpox. About 100 years later, Pasteur introduced vaccines against anthrax and rabies based upon attenuated virulent organisms. The discovery by von Behring in 1890, that serum antibodies could neutralize diphtheria toxin opened the door for a new avenue of vaccine development and passive therapy, whereby preformed antibodies were transferred to at-risk patients. By the beginning of the 20th century, serum obtained from immunized animals was used to treat a variety of diseases including diphtheria and tetanus. The use of human serum followed shortly thereafter in 1907.

Since the turn of the century, a wide range of vaccines and antisera have been introduced to manage infectious and noninfectious diseases (Tab. 1-1). The "first generation" of vaccines were composed of crude detoxified bacterial toxins (diphtheria and tetanus) or killed inactivated preparations of intact bacterial cells (cholera and typhoid fever) or virus (smallpox). Surprisingly, many of these vaccines are still in use and remain essentially unchanged from when first introduced. In the case of diphtheria and tetanus toxoid vaccines, there has been little impetus to modify existing vaccines due to their long history of safety and efficacy. Killed whole cell vaccines (cholera, typhoid fever and pertussis) have always suffered from a safety standpoint and are currently being replaced by a new generation of vaccines.

Tab. 1-1 Currently available vaccines and immunoglobulins.

Type of vaccine or immunoglobulin	Disease
Vaccines	
— bacterial vaccines	Cholera
	Diphtheria
	Haemophilus influenzae b
	Meningococcal meningitis
	Pertussis
	Streptococcus pneumoniae
	Tetanus
	Tuberculosis
	Typhoid fever

— viral vaccines	Hepatitis B
	Influenza
	Japanese encephalitis
	Measles
	Mumps
	Polio
	Rabies
	Rift Valley fever
	Rubella
	Smallpox
	Tick-borne encephalitis
	Varicella
	Yellow fever
Immunoglobulins	
— against bacterial diseases	Diphteria
	Gas gangrene
	H. influenzae, meningococcal meningitis, *Streptococcus pneumoniae* (polyvalent preparation)
	Pertussis
	Pseudomonas aeruginosa
	Tetanus
— against viral diseases	Cytomegalovirus
	Hepatitis A
	Hepatitis B
	Human immunodeficiency virus (HIV) (normal intravenous immunoglobulin preparation administered to HIV-positive infants)
	Measles
	Mumps
	Rabies
	Rubella
	Vaccinia
	Varicella
— against noninfectious diseases	Hypogammaglobulinemia
	Rhesus factor
	Idiotypic thrombocytopenia purpura

Although the past several decades have seen the introduction of several new or improved vaccines against a variety of diseases, such as measles, mumps, rubella, meningococcal meningitis, pneumococcal diseases, typhoid fever, *Haemophilus influenzae* b, varicella, and hepatitis B, there still remains a large number of diseases for which vaccines are needed. A list of these diseases is shown in Tab. 1-2.

Tab. 1-2 Infectious diseases of major public health concern for which no vaccines are currently available.

Acquired Immunodeficiency Syndrome (AIDS)
Escherichia coli diarrhea
Hepatitis A
Leprosy
Malaria
Respiratory Syncytial Virus
Rotavirus
Shigellosis
Shistosomiasis

1.2 Principles and Definitions

1.2.1 Antigens

An antigen is any molecule capable of eliciting either an immune response (either humoral, i.e. antibody-mediated, or cellular, i.e. cell-mediated), or an immune reaction, such as an allergic response [1]. An antigen that evokes an immune response is commonly referred to as an **immunogen**. Only foreign or "non-self" molecules are immunogenic. Usually the larger and more complex a molecule is, the more immunogenic it will be. For example, the gram-negative bacterial cell envelope shown in Fig. 1-1 contains many different somatic (cell-associated) antigens, such as lipopolysaccharide (LPS), outer-membrane proteins and phospholipids. Numerous factors determine the immunogenicity of a purified molecule. Size is of critical importance: proteins with a molecular mass of ≤ 20 000 are poorly immunogenic. Similarly, simple polysaccharides composed of a limited number of repeating monosaccharides are not immunogenic unless their molecular mass exceeds 500 000. Small molecules can be rendered immunogenic by covalently coupling them to larger molecules, forming conjugates.

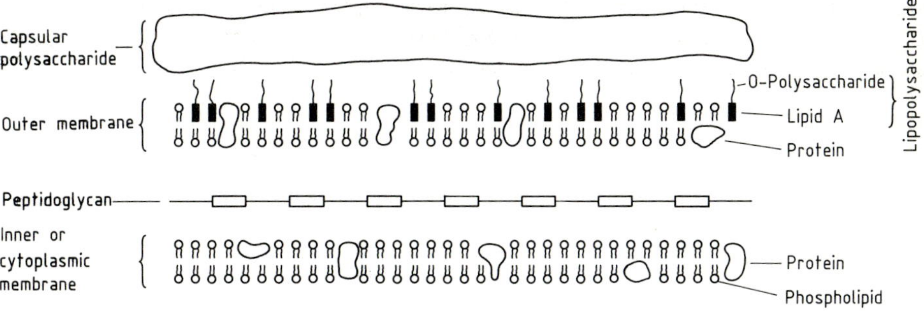

Fig. 1-1 Schematic representation of the Gram-negative bacterial cell envelope.

A single antigen may contain many epitopes, which are specific areas of the molecule with a three-dimensional configuration that induces an immune response or will bind an antibody [1, 2]. Complex molecules, such as large proteins composed of many different amino acids, contain more epitopes than a comparatively simple polysaccharide composed of two or three monosaccharide repeats. The immune response to a given antigen can vary greatly among species due to immune regulation (IR) genes.

The ability of an individual to mount an immune response to a given antigen or type of antigen is controlled by IR genes. For example, native American Indians respond poorly to bacterial polysaccharide antigens [3]. Similarly, people of Hispanic decent also produce lower levels of antibody to several bacterial vaccines as compared to Caucasians [4]. Blood group type also appears to influence the magnitude of the humoral immune response [4].

1.2.2 Antibodies

Antibodies are proteins found primarily in the serum which are produced by B cells (see below) in response to their contact with a foreign antigen. There are several different classes of antibodies with characteristic functions (see Chapter 5, Tab. 5-1). A schematic of an **immunoglobulin G** (IgG) molecule is shown in Fig. 1-2. Immunoglobulins are composed of light and heavy chains held together by disulfide bonds. Each chain has a variable and a constant region [1, 2]. The tertiary structure of the variable region accounts for the specificity of the antibody binding. An antibody produced from a given clone of B cells (see below) recognizes and binds to a given epitope or closely related epitopes. Antibodies which recognize more than one epitope are termed **cross-reactive**. The strength with which an antibody binds to an antigen is termed **affinity** and is determined by the "fit" between the immunoglobulin binding site and the epitope.

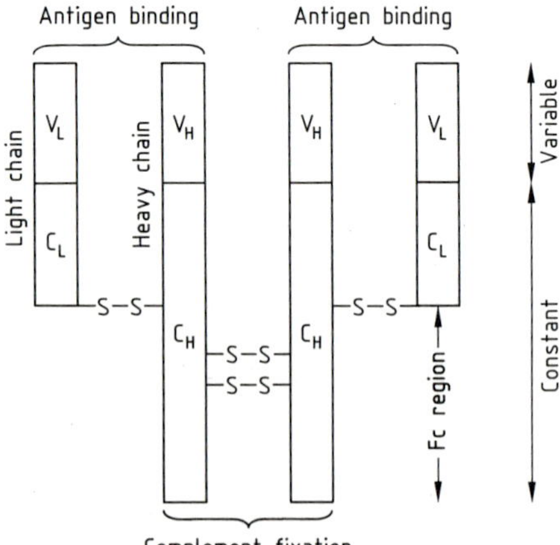

Fig. 1-2 Schematic representation of an immunoglobulin G (IgG) molecule.

Antibodies produced by a single clone of B cells are termed **monoclonal antibodies** and recognize only a single epitope (see Chapter 6). **Polyclonal antibodies** are produced by several B cell clones which recognize the same antigen, but are specific for different epitopes.

Immunoglobulins are divided into five classes termed IgG, IgM, IgA, IgD and IgE based upon physical and structural differences; they are all glycoproteins [1, 2]. The vast majority of immunoglobulins circulates in the plasma fraction, but certain cells of the immune system can express immunoglobulin on their cell surfaces.

Immunoglobulin G (IgG) has a molecular mass of 150 000 dalton and has two antigen binding sites; it represents approximately 80 % of all immunoglobulins in normal serum (8-16 mg/ml). Four IgG subclasses (IgG_1-IgG_4) account for ca. 70, 19, 8 and 3 % of total IgG, respectively. They differ with respect to their antigenic properties in the constant region of the heavy chains. IgG has two antigen binding sites. The functional attributes of these subclasses are detailed in Chapter 5, pp. 100, Tab. 5-1. Immunoglobulin G readily crosses the placenta and provides protection against a variety of infectious diseases in the neonate. For example, immunization of the mother against tetanus shortly before delivery ensures a protective level of antibody for the infant. Immunoglobulin G also diffuses into the extravascular tissue more readily than other immunoglobulin classes. The IgG antibody is thought to be responsible for neutralizing the majority of bacterial toxins (e.g., tetanus and diphtheria toxins) formed during an infection. Upon binding with invading bacteria, IgG activates the complement system (a group of interacting serum proteins) which attracts phagocytic cells. The binding of complement components to the Fc region of IgG allows for the uptake and killing of the bacteria by phagocytes.

Immunoglobulin M is a 900 000 dalton pentamer whose 5 IgG-like units are held together by intramolecular disulfide bonds and stabilized by a polypeptide "anchor" termed the "J-chain". IgM comprises 5-10 % of normal circulating immunoglobulins (1-2 mg/ml). Due to its large size, IgM is confined to the intravascular space.

It binds complement but, unlike IgG, does not bind directly to phagocytic cells. Immunoglobulin M is usually the first antibody class formed in response to foreign antigen exposure. Due to its multivalency, IgM is extremely efficient at agglutinating bacteria. This phenomenon is an important mechanism in the control of bacteremia and the neutralization of LPS released by Gram-negative bacteria.

Immunoglobulin A (IgA) occurs as 160 000 dalton monomers or 320 000 dalton dimers. Monomers are found primarily in the intravascular space and comprise approximately 10-15 % (1.4-4 mg/ml) of total serum immunoglobulins. There are two subclasses, IgA_1 and IgA_2. Dimeric IgA, termed **secretory IgA**, is formed by noncovalent interactions with the "secretory piece", a glycoprotein of about 60 000 daltons. Secretory IgA is the predominant immunoglobulin found in mucous secretions, such as tears, colostrum, pulmonary, intestinal, and genitourinary fluids. IgA can bind complement and react with phagocytic cells.

Although parenteral immunization stimulates a vigorous serum IgA response, secretory IgA is considered to be of greater importance due to its "first line" defensive role in bodily secretions. Secretory IgA plays a critical role in providing protection against respiratory, intestinal, and genitourinary tract pathogens.

Immunoglobulin D (IgD) is a monomer of ca. 180 000 dalton; concentrations vary widely in humans ranging from 0 to ca. 0.4 mg/ml. Compared to other immunoglobulin classes, IgD is very susceptible to proteolysis and possesses a short half-life (about 3 days). Since IgD does not fix complement or bind to phagocytic cells, it is not considered to be a "protective" immunoglobulin as are IgA, IgG and IgM. However, IgD is abundant on the surface of B lymphocytes and may play a central role in the activation process which leads to the development of antibody-secreting plasma cells.

Immunoglobulin E (IgE) is a monomer of 200 000 dalton; its average serum concentration (ca. 250 ng/ml) is the lowest of any immunoglobulin. Although IgE does not fix complement or react directly with phagocytic cells, it has a very high affinity for mast cells and basophils. Immunoglobulin E appears to mediate both a protective and detrimental immune response. At the mucous membrane surface, pathogens or allergens binding to IgE stimulate an acute inflammatory response by triggering the release of potent mediators from mast cells and basophils. A protective role for IgE is indicated in several chronic parasitic infections, most notably schistosomiasis (see Chapter 4) where high levels (> 100 μg/ml) of serum IgE have been noted. Immunoglobulin E induces an inflammatory response and "recruits" effector cells to the area. In contrast, IgE-mediated degranulation of effector cells leads to the release of vasoreactive molecules. Individuals suffering from certain types of allergies can also have elevated serum IgE levels.

1.2.3 Immune Response

The chain of events leading to the formation of an immune response is extremely complicated and not yet completely understood. A minimal model is shown in Fig. 1-3. Humans are capable of forming an immune response to thousands of foreign antigens. The humoral (antibody-mediated) response depends on the **B-cells**, which are lymphocytes derived from bone marrow stem cells. Upon maturation, B cells form antibody-secreting **plasma cells.**

Each clone of B cells has an immunoglobulin molecule with a specific antigen recognition site on its surface. Binding of the appropriate antigen to the B cell causes proliferation of the clone whereby progeny cells secrete antibody whose specificity is identical to that of the cell-surface immunoglobulin. A foreign antigen can be taken up by macrophages, processed and presented upon the cell surface, or may remain in a soluble state. All antigens can be termed T-dependent or T-independent depending on whether they require or do not require the interaction of T cells for antibody synthesis (T cells are lymphocytes derived from the thymus). In the case of a **T-independent antigen** (usually polymers, such as bacterial capsular polysaccharides), the antigen can crosslink the B cell surface antibody molecules of the B cell; this initiates proliferation and antibody snythesis. A **T-dependent antigen** requires, in addition to binding to B cell surface immunoglobulin, the release of T cell factors which act upon the B cell to initiate proliferation [5].

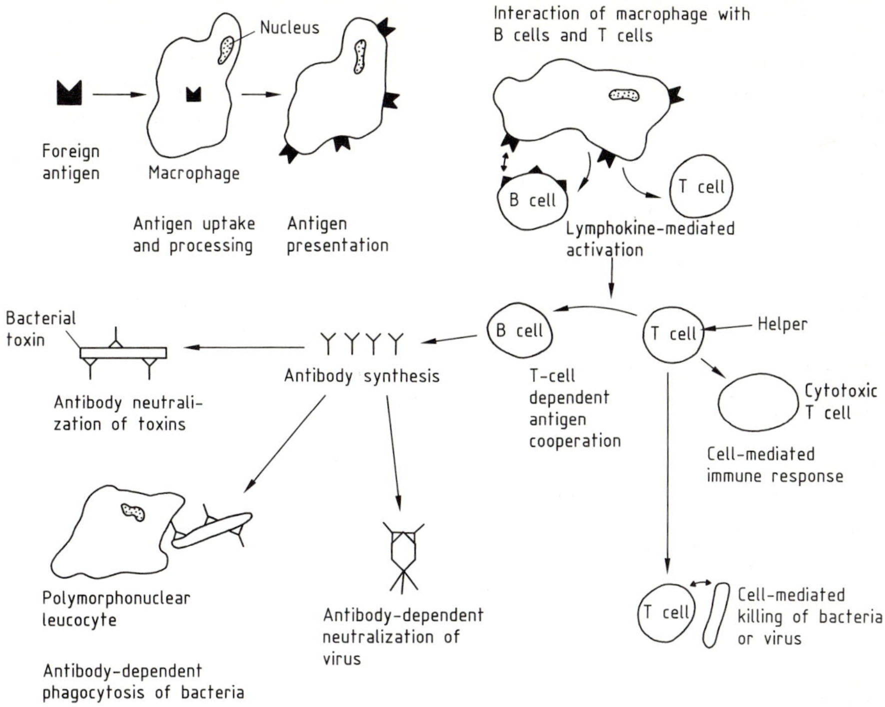

Fig. 1-3 Immunological response cascade to a foreign antigen or vaccine, leading to antibody response or cell-mediated response.

A human exposed to an antigen in this way is considered **primed**. This is a critical factor in immunization. After initial exposure to a T-dependent antigen by immunization, the induced serum antibody concentration is low and returns to near-basal levels comparatively quickly (the average half-life of IgG is ca. 22 days, whereas that of IgM is ca. 5 days). Upon revaccination (boostering) or natural exposure to the pathogen or toxin, a vigorous antibody response rapidly occurs in which high antibody levels are synthesized over a longer period of time. This is termed an **anamnestic response.** Therefore, high levels of serum antibodies do not necessarily have to be present for the individual to be protected by prior vaccination. A T-independent antigen does not usually evoke an anamnestic response.

In general, IgG antibody levels engendered by T-independent antigens tend to remain above baseline levels longer than those induced by T-dependent antigens. Antibody levels to certain bacterial polysaccharide antigens can remain elevated for 5 years or longer after a single vaccination. Although the precise reason for this is not known, it has been postulated that T-independent antigens are resistant to degradation in the body due to their chemical characteristics and are, therefore, cleared slowly. This may allow them to stimulate the immune system for a long period of time.

The induction of a **cell-mediated immune (CMI) response** is rather more complicated and less well defined [1, 2, 5, 6]. The CMI response plays a critical role in immunity to pathogens able to live and proliferate within host cells. The first step is "activation" of T cells. Like B cells, T cells also recognize specific antigens. Recognition of an antigen on the surface of a macrophage by T cells results in the release of **interleukin 1** (IL-1), a lymphokine which activates them. One subpopulation of T cells synthesizes **interleukin 2** (IL-2), also known as T cell growth factor, which causes a second subpopulation of activated T cells expressing the IL-2 receptor to proliferate and become cytotoxic T cells. Cytotoxic T cells recognize the specific antigen they are directed against when this is expressed on the surface of infected cells; thus, they kill infected cells by lysis. A third subpopulation of T cells evolve to be "primed" memory cells which undergo rapid proliferation upon reexposure to the same antigen.

Immunization with a given vaccine may induce either a CMI or a humoral antibody response, or both depending upon the infecting pathogen. Both types of immunity are usually desirable and may act synergistically. For example, vaccine-induced immunity to many viral diseases, such as rabies, measles, mumps and rubella, is confirmed by measuring serum antibody levels. However, infected cells can only be destroyed by cytotoxic T cells. Circulating antibody probably prevents the spread of virus, while cytotoxic T cells eliminate already infected cells. Tuberculosis vaccines which stimulate a good antibody response are less protective than those that produce a poor response due to the suppression of the CMI response, which is critical for protection.

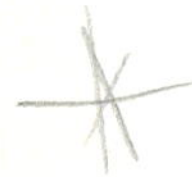

1.2.4 Active Immunization

Active immunization entails the administration of an antigen or antigens to a host in an attempt to elicit a protective immune response. This is the most practical form of immunization in that an individual can be rendered immune to a variety of diseases; in many instances, immunity is life-long. Most vaccines are administered to infants or young children. The trend is to combine monovalent vaccines (composed of a single antigen or vaccine strain) to form multivalent vaccines capable of simultaneously inducing immunity to several diseases. Therefore, infants are routinely immunized against diphtheria, tetanus and pertussis by combining all these vaccines into a single injection. In some countries, inactivated polio is also added to yield a quadrivalent vaccine. Similarly, young children are immunized simultaneously with measles, mumps and rubella vaccine. The ability of the immune system to recognize and respond to a variety of antigens allows this practice to be successful. Combining vaccines which should be administered at the same age allows for less visits to health care centers, a critical point in developing countries where it is often impossible to obtain access to a child over a long period of time to administer vaccines.

Historically, most vaccines have been administered by the parenteral route (i.e. injected with a syringe and needle). This has been an extremely successful approach if the disease is a systemic one, such as diphtheria or measles. However, where the disease is localized, as in the case of intestinal infections such as cholera, parenteral vaccines are of limited use since the immune system at the site of infection (e.g., local immune system) needs to be stimulated [7]. Therefore, a substantial effort is now being concentrated at controlling infectious intestinal diseases through the use of orally administered vaccines. Such vaccines can consist of killed intact bacteria, toxoids (whereby toxins are rendered biologically inactive by treatment with a chemical or heat which maintains their immunogenicity), subunit vaccines, in which only the nontoxic portion of a molecule is used, or live-attenuated vaccines, whereby a strain of virus or bacteria has been rendered nonpathogenic (for example, by passaging virus in cell culture or deletion of bacterial genes), but is still able to multiply to a limited degree, thereby eliciting a protective immune response in the absence of disease symptoms [8].

One major problem with the use of highly purified antigens or subunit vaccines is reduced immunogenicity. Unfortunately, as protective antigens are purified from either bacteria, viruses, or parasites in order to free them from toxic substances such as LPS, their ability to evoke an immune response is reduced. One method by which their immunogenicity can be increased is by the use of an adjuvant, a chemical or carrier substance. Adjuvants function either to present the antigen to the immune system for a prolonged period of time, or to nonspecifically stimulate the immune system by releasing immune modulators, such as lymphokines. To date, only aluminium gels have been licensed as adjuvants for human use. For example, tetanus or diphtheria toxoid is absorbed onto the gel which allows the toxoid to persist longer at the injection site. Several experimental adjuvants, such as monophosphoryl lipid A or derivatives of the immunostimulating peptide termed muramyl dipeptide (MDP), have shown promise in preliminary clinical testing. At present, biologically active peptides, capable of nonspecifically stimulating the immune system via lymphokine release or down-regulating the suppressor arm of the immune system, are being evaluated.

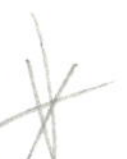

1.2.5 Passive Immunization

Passive immunization entails the transfer of preformed immunoglobulins to a host. In most instances, passive immunity is employed after known or suspected exposure to a given pathogen (for example, after being bitten by a rabid animal). Passive immunization is used in cases where disease progress is rapid unless the pathogen or toxin is neutralized. In such instances, the time needed for the host to mount a protective immune response following vaccination (normally 7-14 days) is too long. In some instances, globulin may be passively transferred as a prophylactic measure as in the case of travellers entering in an area where hepatitis A is endemic.

Such immunoglobulin preparations are assayed to confirm that they contain a high titer of neutralizing antibodies. Such "hyperimmune" globulins must contain at least 5-fold higher levels than normal globulin and are produced by screening plasma units (human) for a given antibody. Alternatively, volunteers may be vaccinated to enrich their plasma for a given antibody.

Currently, immunoglobulin is administered either intramuscularly or intravenously [9]. The amount of globulin that can be given intramuscularly is limited by volume considerations. Intravenous administration allows for comparatively large quantities of immunoglobulin (up to 1 g of immunoglobulin/kg body weight) to be administered quickly [9].

There are several problems related to the preparation of immunoglobulin for passive therapy. The first concerns supply. Identification of plasma donors who are "hyperimmune" to a given antigen requires screening programs which are rather expensive and tedious. Secondly, there exists the possibility of transferring several viral diseases, such as hepatitis B and non-A, non-B hepatitis, with the use of immunoglobulins. Additional screening procedures must be instituted to rule out these possibilities.

An alternative to antibody obtained from donors is the use of human monoclonal antibodies (humabs; see Chapter 6). Humabs can be synthesized by hybridoma cell lines produced by fusing a human B cell secreting a desired antibody to a non-secreting heteromyeloma cell line. Such a hybridoma can be grown in fermentors of up to 1 000 liters in serum-free medium. Antibody yields can reach 100 mg of antibody per liter. The use of humabs can circumvent the need to obtain plasma from many donors and the risk of viral disease transmission, all at a lower cost. Humabs against a variety of infectious agents, such as cytomegalovirus, and diphtheria and tetanus toxins, have been produced and will undergo testing in the near future.

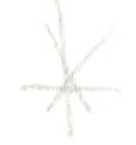

1.2.6 Genetic Engineering

The application of recombinant DNA technology to the field of vaccine development has led to remarkable progress over the past decade. Using such techniques, it is now possible to define critical protective antigenic determinants. These antigens can then be cloned, produced in high quantities by using an appropriate expression system (vector and host), and purified. The first genetically engineered vaccine for human use is against hepatitis B where the surface antigen was cloned, produced in yeast and purified to homogeneity. These vaccines have all but replaced the first generation plasma-derived antigen vaccines due to increased safety and lower costs.

Although numerous live-attenuated vaccines are licensed for use (measles, polio, mumps, rubella, varicella and typhoid fever), these have been derived through rather empirical techniques, such as passage on tissue culture or chemical mutagenesis. Surprisingly, the precise genetic alterations which render these strains avirulent are unknown.

At present, several live-attenuated bacterial vaccine strains have been developed using genetic engineering. The most advanced, in regards to clinical testing, are for cholera and typhoid fever [10, 11]. These strains have been attenuated by inactivating a gene or genes essential for virulence. A related approach has been to clone a given protective antigen and express it in a suitable, nonvirulent "carrier" strain. For example, surface glycoprotein from HIV-1 and rabies virus have been introduced into vaccinia virus (smallpox vaccine). In addition, antigens from several enteric pathogens such as *Shigella sonnei, S. dysenteriae* and *Vibrio cholerae* have been introduced into the licensed live-oral typhoid vaccine strain, Ty21a [10, 11]. Such recombinant strains may prove useful as "bivalent" vaccines, conferring protection against two enteric pathogens.

1.2.7 Practical Considerations for Vaccine Usage

The availability of safe and effective vaccines does not necessarily mean that they will be used to their full benefit. The implementation of vaccination programs can be greatly complicated by a number of factors including (I) economics; (II) perception of the need for vaccination by the public and the medical profession; (III) liability issues; and (IV) the logistics of administering the vaccine. The relative importance of these issues varies depending upon whether the vaccines are to be used in developed or underdeveloped areas of the world.

In underdeveloped nations, the vast majority of vaccines are provided primarily by international agencies such as UNICEF or the Pan American Health Organization, and are aimed at providing the essential childhood immunizations (diphtheria, tetanus, pertussis (DPT), measles, and tuberculosis). Cost is, of course, a major consideration. However, of equal concern is the proper storage and distribution of the vaccine. Even today, a substantial proportion of children do not receive the recommended 3 doses of DPT due to logistical problems.

In developed countries, vaccine "uptake" has been markedly improved by laws which require children to produce documentation that they have been properly immunized before entering primary school. The utilization of adult vaccines (influenza, hepatitis B and pneumococcal vaccine) is largely a matter of perception by the public and medical community. Recently, it has been estimated that less than 30 % of health care workers, for whom vaccination against hepatitis B is recommended, have received the vaccine. Initially, this was due to a combination of concern over the safety of the plasma-derived vaccine and the lack of proper information about the benefits of vaccination. With the introduction of a recombinant vaccine, under-utilization is perceived primarily as an educational issue. Similarly, a relatively small proportion of the aged or infirm are routinely vaccinated against influenza or pneumococcal pneumonia.

Vaccine uptake can also be dramatically influenced by the public view concerning safety. Concern over the safety of the whole-cell pertussis vaccine propagated primarily through the popular press led to a dramatic drop in vaccine use in Japan, Sweden and England during the 1970's, which resulted in several epidemics. This prompted a marked increase in vaccine utilization with a subsequent decline in disease.

1.3 References

1. Roitt, I., Essential Immunology, Fifth edition. Blackwell Scientific Publications, Oxford, U. K., (1984).
2. Davis, B. D., Dulbecco, R., Eisen, H. N., and Ginsberg, H. S., Microbiology: Including Immunology and Molecular Genetics, Third edition. Harper and Row, Publishers, Inc., Hagerstown, MD, (1980).
3. Ambrosino, D. M., Shiffman, G., Gotschlich, E. C., Schur, P. H., Rosenberg, G. A., DeLange, G. G., van Loghem, E., and Siber, G. R., *J. Clin. Invest.* (1985), **75**, 1935.
4. Cryz, S. J., Jr., Fürer, E., Fredeking, T., Cross, A. S., Sadoff, J. C., and Que, J. U., *Lancet* (1989), **i**, 1533.
5. Schwartz, R. H., Yano, A., and Paul, W. E., *Immunol. Rev.,* (1978), **40**, 153.
6. Yamamura, T., and Tada, T., Progress in Immunology V. Academic Press, Tokyo, (1984).
7. Stroler, W., Hanson, L. A., and Sell, K. W. (eds.). Recent Advances in Mucosal Immunity. Raven Press, New York, (1982).
8. Robbins, J. B., Hill, J. C., and Sadoff, J. C. (eds.). Bacterial Vaccines. Seminars in Infectious Dease. Vol. IV. Thieme-Stratton, Inc., New York, (1982).
9. Nydegger, U. E. (ed.). Immunoterapy. A Guide to Immunoglobulin Prophylaxis and Therapy. Academic Press, London, (1981).
10. Levine, M. M., Kaper, J. B., Herrington, D., Ketley, J., Losonsky, G., Tacket, C. O., Tall, B., and Cryz, S. J., CVD 103 and *Lancet* (1988), **2**, 467-470.
11. Black, R. E., Levine; M. M., Clements, M. L., Losonsky, G., Herrington, D., Berman, S., and Formal, S. B., *J. Infect. Dis.* (1987), **155**, 1260-1265.

2. Bacterial Vaccines

S. J. Cryz, Jr.

2.1 Diphtheria Vaccine

Etiological Agent and Pathogenesis. The causative agent of diphtheria is *Corynebacterium diphtheriae*, a Gram-positive non-spore-forming rod, first isolated by Loeffler in 1884. The disease is spread by inhalation of infected droplets. The infecting bacteria colonize the throat. Release of a potent toxin (diphtheria toxin) results in localized tissue necrosis characterized by an inflammatory exudate which can form a pseudomembrane on the posterior pharynx of the nasopharyngeal area. Disease symptoms are due exclusively to the production of diphtheria toxin, a potent inhibitor of eucaryotic protein synthesis, which is spread from the site of infection via the bloodstream. Death is due to the inhibition of protein synthesis by the toxin in various vital organs [1]. Recovery from disease is frequently accompanied by cardiac and/or neurological sequela due to toxin-mediated tissue damage.

History of Immunization Against Diphtheria. Studies by Roux and Yersin in 1888 first demonstrated that diphtheria is a "toxicosis". Two years later, Behring and Kitasato established that the disease could be prevented in animals by immunization with a crude diphtheria toxoid. Initial attempts to extend these findings to humans used a "toxoid" prepared by combining diphtheria toxin and antitoxin. The first large scale immunization program with such a product was performed in New York school children in 1922. Soon after, crude toxoids prepared by formalin treatment of *C. diphtheriae* filtrates replaced toxin-antitoxin toxoids. Routine mass vaccination against diphtheria was initiated in Western Europe and North America shortly after World War II.

Production and Characteristics of Current Diphtheria Vaccine. Diphtheria toxoid is prepared by detoxification of diphtheria toxin with formaldehyde. Derivatives of the hypertoxinogenic Park Williams 8 strain are used by most manufacturers. Large quantities of toxin are produced in fermentors (~ 200-5000 l) where yields of toxin approach 500 mg/l. Although manufacturing processes vary, most employ the following steps. Formalin (0.4-0.6 %) is added to cell-free culture supernatants which are then stored at 35 °C-37 °C for 3 to 5 weeks. Detoxification is accomplished first by reaction of formalin with the ε-amino groups of lysine and then by forming irreversible methylene bridges among available aromatic amino acids. Upon confirmation of detoxification by animal testing, the toxoid is purified by a combination of diafiltration, ammonium sulfate or ethanol fractionation, and anion-exchange chromatography.

Current Immunization Recommendations. Diphtheria toxoid is rarely used as a monovalent vaccine, but is usually combined with tetanus toxoid (DT), pertussis vaccine (DPT), or inactivated polio vaccine (DPT-Pol) adsorbed to aluminium-containing salts which serve as an adjuvant. Toxoid content is usually expressed in Lf (limit of flocculation) with 1 Lf equal to ~ 2 μg of toxoid. For primary immunization of infants, ~ 25 Lf of toxoid is administered intramuscularly starting at 6-12 weeks of age. Three doses are usually administered at 4-8 week intervals with a fourth dose give 4-12 months after the third dose. To maintain life-long immunity, booster doses, together with tetanus toxoid, are recommended every 7-10 years.

To determine the immune status of an individual, a "Schick" test is performed. A minute amount of diphtheria toxin is injected intradermally. A "Schick"-positive reaction is characterized by a central area of necrosis surrounded by an area of erythematous swelling and tenderness due to an insufficient amount of circulating antitoxin (< 0.01 IU/ml) to neutralize the toxin. The reaction is maximal by day 5. Caution must be used in the interpretation of the "Schick" test due to possible allergic reactions against diphtheria toxin which reach a maximum by day 2-3. To rule this out, a separate intradermal injection of diphtheria toxoid (0.005 Lf) should be given simultaneously in a different location. Persons showing a hypersensitivity reaction in the "Schick" test should not be re-immunized as the amount of test antigen is sufficient to stimulate an anamnestic response.

Adverse Reactions. The absolute rate of reactogenicity of diphtheria toxoid is difficult to determine since it is usually administered with tetanus toxoid and pertussis vaccine.

Overall, the vaccine is considered to be safe and to evoke primarily local reactions which are mild and transient.

Vaccine Efficacy. No large scale field trials have ever been performed to determine vaccine efficacy. This is due to the fact that it would be unethical to withhold the vaccine given the dramatic decrease in disease following immunization in the 1920's. Furthermore, there is an overwhelming body of data to indicate that proper use of the vaccine, e.g., a complete immunization regimen, can provide absolute protection against disease. For example, mass vaccination with diphtheria toxoid in Romania in 1958 showed that within 7 years morbidity and mortality due to diphtheria declined to less than 1 % of that seen in 1958. In Western Europe and North America, where vaccination is universal, diphtheria has been virtually eradicated [2]. Rare cases which are seen occur almost exclusively in individuals who lack a proper history of vaccination and, therefore, possess nonprotective levels of antitoxin.

Future Prospects. Given the combination of vaccine safety, efficacy, and cost, there has been little impetus to develop and test a "second generation" diphtheria toxoid. Any such vaccine would have to completely eliminate the possibility of toxic reversion and be more economical to produce. Recent advances have brought these goals into the realm of possibility. Synthetic peptides expressing key epitopes of diphtheria toxin conjugated to carrier proteins can elicit neutralizing antibodies [3]. The drawback with this approach is the cost of purifying the carrier protein, and production of the conjugate.

The most promising new approach to toxoid development is the use of nontoxic mutant proteins, referred to as CRM's [4], derived by recombinant DNA technology. It is now possible to construct such proteins by deletion of specific regions responsible for toxicity [5]. In addition, these "toxoids" can be synthesized in yields equal to that obtained by the current production strains of *C. diphtheriae*. The efficacy of such proteins is currently being evaluated.

2.2 Tetanus Vaccine

Etiological Agent and Pathogenesis. The causative agent of tetanus is the Gram-positive anaerobic spore-forming bacillus, *Clostridium tetani*. The disease, first described by Hippocrates, is contracted via contamination of wounds or abrasions with soil containing *C. tetani* spores or by improper severing of the umbilical cord (neonatal tetanus). Bacteria multiplying at the wound site, often with no overt signs of infection, release a potent protein neurotoxin (tetanus toxin). Tetanus toxin acts upon the central nervous system (CNS) causing spastic paralysis, presumably by interfering with the release of inhibitory neurotransmitters [6]. The toxin enters the bloodstream from the localized site of infection and gains access to the CNS. The majority of tetanus cases are currently found in neonates due to the unsterile severing of the umbilical cord.

History of Vaccination Against Tetanus. The identification of tetanus as a toxicosis by Faber in 1890 led to the development of crude tetanus toxoids as early as 1893. Initial attempts to vaccinate against tetanus were carried out during World War I. By 1926, parenteral immunization of humans with a safe and effective formalin toxoid was achieved. Until the mid-1960's, only such crude toxoids were available.

Production and Characteristics of Current Tetanus Vaccine. The presently used tetanus toxoid is a partially purified preparation. The hypertoxinogenic Harvard strain of *C. tetani* is most widely used for production of tetanus toxin. The bacteria are grown in fermentors until the cells autolyse, thereby releasing the toxin into the medium. Intact cells are removed by filtration. Formalin is added to the filtrate to a final concentration of 0.4 %-0.6 %, the pH adjusted to between 7.4 and 7.6, and the mixture held at 35°C-37°C for about 4 weeks. After confirmation of detoxification by animal testing, tetanus toxoid is purified by diafiltration and ammonium sulfate fractionation.

Current Immunization Recommendations. Tetanus toxoid is most frequently adsorbed to an aluminium salt-adjuvant and administered together with diphtheria toxoid (DT), pertussis vaccine (DPT), or inactivated polio vaccine (DPT-Pol). For primary immuization of infants, each dose of vaccine contains 20-30 Lf's of tetanus toxoid as DPT or DPT-Pol. Immunization starts at 6-12 weeks of age and consists of 3 doses given at 4-8 week intervals with a fourth dose given 4-12 months later. To maintain life-long immunity ($\geq$ 0.01 IU/ml of serum), booster doses often combined together with diphtheria toxoid are recommended every 7-10 years. Tetanus vaccine is often administered as a routine prophylactic measure following puncture wound trauma. This practice can lead to hyperimmunization and attendant reactions. Alternatively, an individual may be "tolerized" by repeated vaccinations and therefore, unable to mount a protective immune response. Therefore, care should be taken to determine a patient's immunization history before deciding upon the administration of a booster. Currently, it is recommended that pregnant women should be vaccinated, with the final dose ~ 3 weeks before expected delivery. The immune response of humans to tetanus vaccine can vary widely among individuals [7]. Antibody production does not necessarily correlate with the amount of tetanus toxoid administered [7]. However, the immunization schedule used appears to influence the magnitude of the immune reaction [8].

Adverse Reactions. Reactions of consequence following vaccination with tetanus toxoid are infrequent. Swelling, pain, and/or redness at the injection site is the most common occurrence. However, immediate and delayed type hypersensitivity and Arthus-like reaction, and in rare instances (˜< 1 case per 2 million injections), neurological sequelae have been noted [6]. The majority of severe reactions are associated with high levels of anti-tetanus antibody. Therefore, close attention should be paid to the interval between booster doses to avoid these occurrences.

Vaccine Efficacy. Data supporting the efficacy of tetanus toxoid vaccine comes primarily from retrospective analysis of attack rates in immune versus nonimmune populations. The first such study was the evaluation of soldiers during World War II where it was found that tetanus occurred primarily in nonimmune individuals. Studies by Newell et al. [9] showed that immunization of pregnant women completely prevented neonatal tetanus. Currently, cases of tetanus observed in the United States occurr exclusively in nonimmune individuals. Numerous studies have also shown that abbreviated 1 or 2 dose immunization regimens are able to induce long-lasting immunity [6]. This is of particular importance in developing countries where a multidose immunization regimen may not be feasible due to an inadequate health care delivery system or economic constraints.

Future Prospects. As with diphtheria toxoid, the current tetanus vaccine has been shown to be an extremely economic, effective, and safe vaccine. Efforts directed to a "new generation" of tetanus vaccine are aimed at providing a toxoid more amenable to mass vaccination. The main thrust has been to produce a safer, more immunogenic toxoid capable of inducing long-lasting immunity after 1 or 2 administrations without reactogenic adjuvants. The substitution of glutaraldehyde for formaldehyde has been shown to yield a safe and immunogenic vaccine not requiring adjuvants [10]. It is also feasible to produce toxoids by recombinant DNA techniques similar to those described for diphtheria toxin [5].

2.3 Pertussis Vaccine

Etiological Agent and Pathogenesis. *Bordetella pertussis*, the cause of pertussis or "whooping cough", is a Gram-negative rod first isolated by Bordet and Gengou in 1906. Man is the only known host for *B. pertussis*. The disease is spread by infectious droplets with the vast majority of cases occurring in young children (≤ 6 years of age). *B. pertussis* shows a marked trophism for the ciliated epithelial cells of the upper respiratory tract. Initial symptoms are similar to that of the common cold, but worsen within 10-20 days. The paraoxysmal stage, lasting an average of 15-20 days, is characterized by severe bouts of coughing. The convalescent stage can last for many months during which time secondary infections can present a major problem. *B. pertussis* remains localized within the upper respiratory tract and can only be isolated during the initial disease stages. This has led to the theory that the severe symptoms seen are toxin-induced [11]. This is supported by the fact that *B. pertussis* can synthesize a large number of toxic extracellular factors including pertussis toxin (also referred to as lymphocytosis promoting factor), adenylate cyclase, dermonecrotic toxin, and tracheal cytotoxin [12].

History of Vaccination Against Pertussis. Attempts at immunization against pertussis were initiated in the 1920s using killed whole-cell vaccines [13]. These studies demonstrated that vaccination could not only prevent a substantial proportion of disease, but that symptoms in vaccinated individuals who became infected were milder than in unvaccinated controls. Routine large scale immunization against pertussis began shortly after World War II using standardized whole-cell vaccines of a known potency. Even though these vaccines have recently been under attack regarding safety issues (see below), they remain in use today in most areas of the world except Japan, where acellular vaccines have been used since 1980 (see below).

Production and Characteristics of Current Pertussis Vaccine. At present, there is no standardized method, culture medium, or bacterial strain used to produce pertussis vaccine. A given manufacturer's production procedure is designed to yield a vaccine which will meet the minimal requirements of the appropriate regulatory agency. *B. pertussis* is usually grown in fermentors on synthetic or semi-synthetic medium. The cells are harvested by centrifugation and resuspended to a given opacity using a reference standard. Inactivation is accomplished by heating, the addition of formalin or thimerosal, or a combination of the above. Given the diversity of production techniques employed, it is important to note that toxic components which escape inactivation can vary considerably from manufacturer to manufacturer.

Current Immunization Recommendations. Pertussis vaccine is used almost exclusively in combination with diphtheria and tetanus vaccines. The vaccine is adsorbed onto an aluminium salt adjuvant. Immunization usually commences at 6-12 weeks of age and consists of 3 doses of vaccine given intramuscularly at 4-8 week intervals with a fourth dose given 4-12 months later. Vaccination with the acellular vaccine currently used in Japan consists of 2-3 doses of vaccine given at 4-8 week intervals starting at 2 years of age.

Adverse Reactions. The majority of children receiving pertussis vaccine will have some type of adverse reaction. Approximately 40-50 % of children will experience a local reaction and 30-40 % a systemic reaction (anorexia, vomiting, fretfulness, fever, or persistent crying) [14]. Of greater concern is the infrequent occurrence of convulsions and hypotonia temporally associated with vaccination. Based upon concerns regarding vaccine safety, a large scale study was initiated in England to determine the incidence of serious reactions in children aged 2-36 months [15]. The risk of vaccine-induced neurological illness was estimated to be 1 per 110 000 vaccinations and that for encephalopathy, 1 per 310 000 vaccinations. It must be noted that establishing a causal relationship in individual cases in such a study is extremely difficult and incidence rates were based on a temporal basis. Further complicating matters is the fact that neurological symptoms believed to be vaccine-related constitute only a small proportion of similar cases seen in this age group. Review of these data by health authorities has led to the conclusion that the benefit of vaccination outweighs the attendant risk given the fact that clinical pertussis can often result in neurological sequela.

Vaccine Efficacy. The first indication of vaccine efficacy came from a trial conducted during an epidemic in 1929 on the Faroe Islands where vaccination afforded 73 % protection against clinical disease [13]. An extensive amount of information has been obtained from surveillance studies in Japan, England, Sweden and the United States where disease incidence has been found to inversely correlate with the overall immune status of the general population. For example, routine immunization against pertussis in the United States has reduced the disease incidence from approximately 150/100 000 in 1940 to less than 40/100 000 in 1966, a level which has remained fairly constant. Even more dramatic has been the drop in mortality rates, from 30/100 000 in 1940 to less than 0.01/100 000 by 1966. While the latter may be attributable in large part to antibiotics and advances in supportive care, there is good data to indicate that the disease is less severe in vaccinated versus nonvaccinated individuals.

Routine immunization against pertussis in Japan was initiated between 1947 and 1949 with an acceptance rate of roughly 90 %. The number of pertussis cases country-wide declined from 152 072 in 1947 to less than 400 by 1971. In 1975, a controversy concerning vaccine safety briefly halted vaccine usage. When it was resumed, the acceptance rate declined to about 25-30 %. Pertussis returned to epidemic proportions by 1979 with more than 13 000 cases reported nationally. At the urging of federal health authorities, vaccine acceptance rates increased to 65-70 % by 1982 with a concomitant decline in cases.

Similarly, concerns of vaccine safety in England resulted in a dramatic decline in vaccine acceptance from ~ 80 % in 1973 to ~ 30 % in 1978. As in Japan, the disease became epidemic with more than 100 000 cases reported between 1977 and 1980. In Sweden routine vaccination against pertussis was initiated in the early 1950's. One decade later, greater than 90 % of children were considered to be immune. Due to changes in the manufacturing technique, the pertussis vaccine used for some time in the mid-1970's was not potent. Shortly after, a marked increase of pertussis cases was seen. When an effective vaccine was reintroduced, the disease incidence was dramatically reduced.

Case-contact studies have shown the whole-cell vaccine to be 63-95 % effective at preventing overt disease. Efficacy of acellular vaccines is discussed below.

Future Prospects. Recent efforts to develop a "second generation" pertussis vaccine have been centered around using purified detoxified antigen preparations containing a minimum amount of lipopolysaccharide (LPS). Several such acellular vaccines have been developed and clinically evaluated. These vaccines are composed of detoxified pertussis toxin (PT) alone or in combination with filamentous hemagglutinin (FHA), two key protective antigens [16]. The first generation acellular vaccines were produced in Japan, whereby supernatant from static cultures was used as a source of antigen. Processing of cell-free supernatants entailed ammonium sulfate precipitation followed by sucrose density gradient ultracentrifugation to simultaneously enrich for PT and FHA and eliminate LPS. PT was inactivated by formalin treatment. Preliminary testing in Japan showed the vaccine to be far better tolerated than whole-cell vaccine. Case-contact studies revealed the vaccine to be ~ 90 % effective. In addition, there has been no increase in pertussis since the introduction of the acellular vaccine.

Second generation acellular vaccines of a greater purity have been produced using fermentor-grown cultures and processing techniques suitable for large scale production. A monovalent formalin PT toxoid and a bivalent PT toxoid-FHA vaccine have been evaluated in a placebo-controlled trial in 5-11 month-olds in Sweden. Children received 2 doses of placebo or vaccine subcutaneously 8-12 weeks apart. The small number of children vaccinated (< 3 000) does not allow for evaluation of vaccine safety regarding the rare neurological reactions. However, the vaccine evoked far fewer local reactions in comparison to the whole-cell vaccine. After 15 months of surveillance, efficacy against culture-confirmed cases of pertussis was 54 % (95 % confidence intervals 26-72 %) for the monovalent toxoid and 69 % (47-82 %) for the two-component vaccine. Protection against severe disease, defined as cough lasting longer than 30 days, was 80 % (59-91 %) and 79 %, respectively [17]. One disconcerting finding was four deaths in the vaccine groups due to invasive bacterial infections, three of which occurred in the group that received the two-component vaccine. There were no deaths from comparable causes in the placebo group. After exhaustive analysis, it was concluded that they could not be attributed to the vaccine [18]. However, the license application for the two-component vaccine has recently been withdrawn over concerns of low vaccine efficacy and safety [19].

Unfortunately, due to trial design, the critical questions of vaccine safety and efficacy as compared to the whole-cell vaccine could not be addressed. In essence, this trial has raised more questions than it has answered. The safety of formalin-inactivated vaccines has been questioned due to the fact that there are no lysine groups in the S_1 subunit of PT which contains the enzymatic active site. Formalin is believed to mediate its detoxifying activity by modification of the ε-amino group of lysine. Also, the need for a whole-cell arm in any future pertussis vaccine trial appears to be critical to answer the question of relative vaccine efficacy.

Several PT toxoids have been developed independent of the use of formalin. A glutaraldehyde-treated preparation has been shown to be safe and immunogenic in 3-6 month-old children. A peroxide-inactivated toxoid has also been found to be safe and immunogenic in adults. Finally, a toxoid produced by treatment with tetranitromethane is safe and immunogenic in adults and in 14-18 month-old children who had received the whole-cell vaccine as infants. It is possible that one or more of these vaccines will be evaluated for efficacy in the near future.

2.4 Typhoid Fever Vaccine

Etiological Agent and Pathogenesis. *Salmonella typhi,* the causative agent of typhoid fever, is a Gram-negative bacillus first isolated by Gaffky in 1884. Infection is due to ingestion of the organisms in contaminated food or water. The bacteria penetrate the epithelium of the small bowel and are ingested by reticuloendothelial cells. Unlike most bacteria, the typhoid bacillus can survive and multiply within phagocytic cells whereby it is disseminated, most notably to the spleen, liver, lymph nodes, and gallbladder. Symptoms appear 1-2 weeks after exposure when the bacteria enter the bloodstream. Even when appropriate treatment is initiated, 1-2 % of those infected will become chronic asymptomatic carriers serving as an infectious reservoir. Typhoid fever is primarily a disease in developing countries or in areas of poor sanitation. In endemic areas, the disease is primarily contracted by school-aged children, but travellers of all ages entering an endemic area are at risk.

History of Vaccination Against Typhoid Fever. Attempts at immunizing man against typhoid fever were initiated as early as 1896. The first mass vaccination effort was conducted by the British Army during World War I using a killed whole-cell vaccine. The attack rate among vaccinated soldiers was far less than among nonimmunized soldiers. Based upon these findings, the use of whole-cell vaccines became a common practice in the armed forces.

In the 1960s and 1970s, several attempts were made to immunize against typhoid fever via the oral route. The first of such studies used killed bacteria which were administered to volunteers at 1 x 10^{11}/dose. Twelve doses resulted in a modest, but significant protection rate of 30 % [20]. Field trials conducted in India between 1968 and 1974 showed that such killed preparations were ineffective at preventing disease.

An alternative approach to oral vaccines against typhoid was to use attenuated live-oral vaccine strains. The first vaccine candidate was a streptomycin-dependent mutant developed by Reitman in 1967 [21]. When orally administered to volunteers in doses of up to 10^{11} bacteria, this strain evoked no adverse reactions. Good levels of protection (66-78 %) were achieved when freshly harvested cultures were used to vaccinate subjects. However, lyophilized preparations afforded little or no protection [21], which diminished interest in this strain.

The second live-oral vaccine candidate, a *gal* ε mutant termed Ty21a, was developed by Germanier and co-workers [22]. Freshly harvested cultures of this strain were found to be safe and effective in volunteer challenge studies [23]. A lyophilized Ty21a preparation given in combination with a liquid buffer was found to afford > 90 % protection for 3 years in a field trial conducted in Cairo, Egypt [24].

Production and Characteristics of Current Typhoid Vaccines. Killed whole-cell vaccines are usually produced from the Ty2 strain of *S. typhi*. Fermentor grown cultures are inactivated either by heating in combination with phenol or formaldehyde or by acetone-drying. Although the latter method has been shown to yield a more efficacious vaccine (see below), only the vaccine produced by the former method is readily available. Each dose of vaccine contains 1-3 x 10^9 killed organisms in 0.5 ml. Vaccine potency is estimated by a mouse-protection test.

The attenuated live-oral Ty21a vaccine strain is produced from fermentor grown cultures. The harvested cells are suspended in a cryoprotective medium and lyophilized. The lyophilizate is placed in gelatin capsules which are then coated with an acid-resistant layer. Each capsule contains 1-5 x 10^9 viable bacteria. Vaccine potency is based upon the number of viable organisms per capsule [25].

Current Immunization Recommendations. Typhoid vaccine is used to immunize individuals living in endemic areas or travellers entering such areas. Two doses of whole-cell vaccine administered subcutaneously or intramuscularly 14 days apart are recommended. A single booster dose is advised for individuals travelling from a non-endemic to an endemic area if 2-3 years have elapsed since primary immunization.

Three doses of attenuated live-oral vaccine are ingested on alternate days. An additional complete immunization course is advised if more than 1-2 years have elapsed since primary immunization when re-entering an endemic area. The vaccine is for use in children 6 years of age and older and in all ages of non-immunocompromised adults.

Adverse Reactions. Reactions following immunization with the parenteral whole-cell vaccine are frequent and can consist of local pain, swelling, and redness, often accompanied by fever, chills, and malaise. Transient debilitating reactions occur in ~ 10 % of vaccine recipients. Due to the high rate of adverse reactions, parenteral typhoid vaccine is not widely used as a public health measure.

Reactions following ingestion of the live-oral Ty21a vaccine are rare (< 1 per 100 000 doses administered). Reactions are usually mild, transient, and resolve of their own accord. Gastrointestinal disturbances and rash have been most frequently reported.

Vaccine Efficacy. To accurately assess the efficacy of parenteral typhoid vaccine, several placebo-controlled field trials were conducted among civilians in the 1960s [26]. In most instances, two doses of either heat-phenol or acetone-dried vaccine were administered. Protection rates ranged from 51-77 % and 79-93 %, respectively, for up to 7 years of observation. A further trial was conducted in Tonga between 1966 and 1973 where school-aged children received 1 or 2 doses of acetone-dried vaccine. Surprisingly, one dose of vaccine gave no protection whereas 2 doses afforded only 40 % protection.

Efficacy of the live oral Ty21a vaccine administered in enteric-coated capsules has been evaluated in double-blind placebo-controlled field trials in school-aged children in Santiago, Chile [27] and Plaju, Indonesia. Three doses of vaccine were found to provide about 70 % protection over a 3-year period [27]. Continued surveillance has shown that high levels (≥ 70 %) of protection extend well into a fourth year [28]. Preliminary results indicate that protection is maintained well into the fifth year post-vaccination.

A field trial conducted in Plaju, Indonesia [29], was designed to address two questions: I) to determine absolute vaccine efficacy in an area with an extremely high attack rate (> 500/100 000 per year); and II) to compare vaccine formulations, the enteric-coated capsules and a liquid formulation, whereby the lyophilized vaccine is reconstituted in a buffer solution immediately prior to ingestion. This field trial site has several characteristics worth mentioning before discussing vaccine efficacy. First, attempts to control typhoid fever in this area by the use of a parenteral vaccine were unsuccessful. Secondly, the vast majority of disease is food-borne since the water supply is clean. This means that the infective dose is comparatively high due to the ability of *S. typhi* to grow to a high density in food.

The study population consisted of individuals from about 3 years to 45 years of age. Three doses of vaccine were administered at weekly (instead of on alternate days) intervals. Efficacy after two years of surveillance was 41 % for the enteric-coated capsules and 55 % for the liquid formulation. This difference was not statistically significant. An interesting, though unexplained phenomenon, was the finding that although immunization afforded good levels (~ 55-65 %) of protection in 3-6 year-olds and in individuals > 17 years of age, efficacy was poor (~ 30 %) in those between the ages of 4 and 16.

A field trial of a similar design was simultaneously conducted in Santiago, Chile. Although the code for this study has yet to be broken, an interim analysis of the data indicated that the liquid formulation afforded significantly higher protection than the enteric-coated formulation. If this trend is maintained after the final analysis, in all likelihood, a liquid formulation will be made commercially available.

Future Prospects. Currently, two additional typhoid vaccines are undergoing clinical evaluation. The first is a double auxotrophic mutant of *S. typhi* requiring ρ-aminobenzoate and adenine [30]. Both a V_1 positive and negative variant (see below) have been isolated. Ingestion of up to 10^{10} organisms elicited no reactions. Immunization engendered a poor humoral immune response to *S. typhi* somatic antigens. However, most vaccines did manifest a specific cell-mediated immune response to *S. typhi* O-antigen [30].

The second candidate vaccine is a *S. typhi* capsular polysaccharide termed V_1. Purified V_1 antigen is safe upon parenteral immunization [31]. This vaccine has been evaluated in Nepal and South Africa [32, 33]. After 17 months of surveillance in Nepal, a single dose of vaccine conferred 72 % protection against culture-confirmed cases of typhoid fever. Similarly, a single dose of vaccine afforded 64 % protection against disease after 21 months of surveillance in South Africa [33]. No data is yet available regarding the long-term protection afforded by this vaccine.

2.5 *Streptococcus pneumoniae* Vaccine

Etiological Agent and Pathogenesis. *Streptococcus pneumoniae*, often referred to as "pneumococcus," is a Gram-positive diplococcus first isolated by Sternberg and Pasteur in 1881. The pneumococcus can be thought of as an opportunistic pathogen, usually causing disease subsequent to a viral infection or in a compromised individual. Pneumonia is the disease syndrome most frequently caused by *S. pneumoniae*. Bacteremia and meningitis are often sequela to pneumococcal pneumonia. *S. pneumoniae* is also a leading cause of otitis media in young children. The pneumococcus often colonizes the nasopharynx of healthy individuals which then serve as infectious foci. The organisms can then spread to another person by infected droplets or translocate to the inner ear or lungs following a viral infection.

History of Vaccination Against Pneumococcal Disease. Early attempts at immunization against pneumococcal pneumonia employed heat-killed whole-cell vaccines (for a review see reference [34]). The majority of these trials yielded equivocal results due to a lack of knowledge regarding the seroepidemiology of disease-causing pneumococci and trial design. However, these trials and related studies led to the conclusion that immunity to pneumococcal disease is mediated by serospecific anti-capsular polysaccharide (anti-CPS) antibody. Felton and co-workers initiated a large scale trial in the mid-1930s using a bivalent CPS vaccine. The results showed a modest decrease in disease in the vaccinated group. Conclusive proof of vaccine efficacy came from vaccine trials conducted by MacLeod et al. [35] and Kaufman using polyvalent vaccines. Protection was serospecific. Further studies showed that vaccines comprising up to six distinct capsular antigens could be effectively used [35]. The first pneumococcal polysaccharide vaccines were hexavalent and were licensed in the early 1950s. However, owing to the belief that antibiotics could effectively control all pneumococcal disease, vaccine acceptance was low, leading to a halt in production.

Production and Characteristics of Currently Available Vaccine. The vaccine licensed for current use is composed of the following 23 types of purified capsular polysaccharide: 1, 2, 3, 4, 5, 6B, 7F, 8, 9N, 9V, 10A, 11A, 12F, 14, 15B, 17F, 18C, 19A, 19F, 20, 22F, 23F and 33F. These antigen types were selected based upon seroepidemiological surveillance studies of bacteremic isolates [36].

Pneumococcal CPS's are purified by a variety of techniques, depending upon serotype, which include precipitation with organic solvents, treatment with detergent, digestion with DNase, RNase and protease and ultracentrifugation. The vaccine contains only trace quantities of protein and nucleic acids (≤ 2 % wt/wt) and is analyzed for a variety of CPS constituents, serological purity, and pyrogenicity. Vaccine potency is based upon the determination of the molecular weight of the CPS's, since immunogenicity in humans is dependent upon those antigens possessing a minimum size. One human dose consists of 25 µg of each antigen in 0.5 ml administered intramuscularly or subcutaneously.

Current Recommendations for Vaccine Usage. Pneumococcal vaccine is currently recommended for immunocompetent individuals with underlying clinical conditions that increase their risk of acquiring pneumococcal bacteremia or pneumonia which include alcoholism, asplenia, sickle-cell anemia, reduced pulmonary function, congestive heart failure, diabetes, reduced renal function, and cirrhosis [37]. It is also felt that routine vaccination of the elderly is warranted due to the increased incidence of disease in this population group. Patients with various underlying conditions (leukemia, Hodgkin's disease, myeloma, and the recipients of immunosuppressive drugs) which render them susceptible to pneumococcal disease may be considered candidates for vaccination even though a proportion may not respond to immunization [37]. Revaccination is not advised due to the severe reactions elicited.

Adverse Reactions. Pneumococcal vaccine is considered to be very safe [37]. Mild local reactions occur in about 30-40 % of vaccinees. Fever and severe local reactions occur in about 1 % of vaccine recipients. Anaphylactic reactions are extremely rare with a frequency of five cases per million doses administered. Severe local and systemic reactions are more likely to occur upon revaccination.

Vaccine Efficacy. Currently, there is considerable controversy concerning the degree of protection provided by pneumococcal vaccine. The vaccine was found to be highly effective at reducing the incidence of pneumococcal pneumonia among South African gold miners [38]. However, this population differs substantially in age and in general health when compared to those patients for which the vaccine is now recommended. Recently, several studies have attempted to accurately determine vaccine efficacy among debilitated and/or elderly patients. Bolan et al. [39] compared the distribution of *S. pneumoniae* serotypes among vaccinated and non-vaccinated individuals with invasive pneumococcal disease. Efficacy was estimated to range from 61-65 %. In contrast, a controlled vaccine trial that included approximately 2 300 high-risk patients, aged 55 or above, did not demonstrate any significant benefit from vaccination [40]. The most likely reason for this finding is the inability of such patients to mount or maintain a protective antibody response following vaccination. Similar findings were reported by Leech et al. [41] in a study of patients suffering from chronic pulmonary disease. In spite of these divergent findings, health authorities still strongly recommend immunization based upon risk-benefit analysis.

Future Prospects. The current pneumococcal vaccine is poorly immunogenic in children under 2 years of age and in certain debilitated patient populations [37]. Attempts have been made to bolster immunogenicity by covalently coupling pneumococcal CPS to carrier proteins [42]. Such conjugates were found to engender a more vigorous response in mice and rhesus monkeys when compared to native CPS [43]. However, a type 6A-tetanus toxoid conjugate administered to young adult volunteers was found to be only slightly more immunogenic than native 6A-CPS, nor did a booster dose significantly increase anti-CPS antibody levels [44]. However, it must be noted that these volunteers had been previously immunized with tetanus toxoid and possessed low, but detectable, levels of antibody to 6A-CPS. It remains to be seen if such pneumococcal conjugate vaccines display increased immunogenicity in children $\leq$ 2 years of age or in debilitated individuals.

2.6 *Shigella* Vaccines

Etiological Agent and Pathogenesis. Shigellosis or bacillary dysentery is caused by various species of *Shigellae,* most notably *S. sonnei, S. flexneri* 2a and 3, and *S. dysenteriae* 1. Disease results from ingestion of the organism. It is estimated that as few as 10 bacteria are sufficient to cause disease in humans, thus making it the most infective bacterial enteric pathogen. In developing countries where the attack rate can exceed 100 000 cases/million population, shigellosis is primarily a disease of young children aged 6 months to 6 years.

Once ingested, the organisms penetrate the intestinal epithelium of the colon and rapidly multiply. This leads to localized inflammation and ulceration, possibly due to synthesis of a potent cytotoxin [45]. Symptoms include fever, bloody diarrhea, cramps, tenesmus, and shock. The mortality rate for untreated disease can exceed 10 %.

History of Vaccine Against Shigellosis. Immunization of humans with killed whole-cell vaccines administered parenterally was found to provide no significant protection against shigellosis [46]. Subsequent attempts at immunization have therefore centered around use of attenuated live oral vaccine strains. Streptomycin-dependent derivatives of *S. flexneri* and *S. sonnei* were evaluated as vaccine candidates. Such vaccines were well tolerated and provide significant immunity for 6-12 months [47, 48]. These vaccines were not pursued further due to the necessity of administering multiple (four) doses for primary immunization, yearly boostering to maintain efficacy and genetic instability.

Formal et al. [49] have sought to produce live oral *Shigella* vaccines by conjugal transfer of genes coding for *S. flexneri* surface antigens into *E. coli.* Multiple doses evoked no significant adverse reactions when fed to volunteers, but failed to protect against subsequent challenge [49].

The identification of critical *Shigellae* protective antigens has allowed for their expression in the attenuated live oral typhoid vaccine strain *S. typhi* Ty21a [50]. One strain, termed *S. typhi* Ty21a-5076-1C, carries a plasmid coding for the Form I (O-polysaccharide) antigen of *S. sonnei.* This strain is safe when administered to volunteers and has afforded significant protection in volunteer studies [51].

Production and Characterization of Current Vaccines. At present, no vaccines are available for use against shigellosis.

Future Prospects. As noted above, *S. typhi* 5076-1C, expressing *S. sonnei* Form I antigen (the O-polysaccharide of LPS), has shown promise in volunteer studies. However, efficacy has been found to vary from lot to lot. Two lots produced from agar plate-grown bacteria were protective, whereas 2 other lots were not. The only identifiable difference was the degree of flagellation, i.e., flagellated lots were more efficacious. In addition, two fermentor-grown lots which lacked flagella were also non-effective. Since large scale production of vaccine using agar-grown cultures is not feasible, attempts have been made to produce highly flagellated fermentor-grown vaccine lots. One such lot was found to offer no significant protection against challenge. The reason for such variable results can not be stated with certainty. One potential reason may be due to the fact that the *S. sonnei* O-PS is not covalently attached to the core of *S. typhi* LPS [52], but rather covers the surface in a manner similar to a capsule. This could have several implications, the most important being the prevention of *S. typhi* from establishing the limited infection necessary to induce a protective immune response. It is known that the serum anti-*S. typhi* LPS antibody response was significantly lower in volunteers receiving the 5076-1C strain compared to Ty21a, indicating an aborted immune response. Another possibility is that it may be essential for the *S. sonnei* O-PS to be covalently attached to the *S. typhi* LPS core to evoke a protective immune response, especially if cell-mediated immunity is critical. Another concern is the relatively poor stability of the *S. sonnei* plasmid in Ty21a. Attempts are now being made to subclone the relevant antigens and to prepare a strain in which the Form I antigen is covalently coupled to an LPS core. Baron and co-workers have recently described the construction of a *S. typhi* Ty21a strain expressing *S. flexneri* 2a type and group antigens [53], This strain has not yet been clinically evaluated.

Genes coding for the production of the O-antigen of *S. dysenteriae* 1 have been cloned and placed on a plasmid [54]. It has been possible to express the *S. dysenteriae* O-antigen in *E. coli* K12, in aromatic amino acid mutants of *S. typhi* and in *S. typhi* Ty21a by introduction of the recombinant plasmid.

Lindberg and co-workers have constructed an aromatic amino acid deficient strain of *S. sonnei* similar to that described above for *S. typhi*. This strain was found to be safe and protective when tested in monkeys. Human studies are planned for the near future.

2.7 Cholera Vaccine

Etiological Agent and Pathogenesis. The causative agent of cholera is *Vibrio cholerae*, a Gram-negative motile bacillus which is transmitted via the fecal-oral route. Upon passage through the stomach acid barrier, *V. cholerae* colonizes the ileum where it rapidly multiplies. The release of a potent enterotoxin (cholera toxin) causes the massive watery diarrhea typical of the disease [55]. In most cases, oral or intravenous fluid replacement is sufficient treatment.

History of Vaccination Against Cholera. Parenteral whole-cell cholera vaccines were employed by Fenan as early as 1885. Starting in the 1960s, several placebo-controlled field trials were performed using inactivated whole-cell vaccines or cholera antigens (see "Vaccine efficacy").

There have been numerous attempts to orally vaccinate against cholera. Freter and Gangarosa [56] demonstrated in 1963 that multiple doses of heat-killed *V. cholerae* administered orally could evoke both a local and humoral antibody response. Cash et al. [57] subsequently showed that 10 daily oral doses of 1.6 x 10^{10} killed vibrios afforded significant protection against a homologous challenge. However, parenteral vaccine gave slightly better protection. Although promising, the massive quantities of organisms used and the need for multiple doses made this approach expensive and cumbersome.

Several environmental isolates of *V. cholerae* with reduced virulence have been evaluated as live-oral vaccines. These strains failed to provide significant protection due to their inability to colonize the small bowel and evoke a protective immune response [58]. A hypotoxinogenic mutant of *V. cholerae* isolated by chemical mutagenesis afforded significant protection against diarrhea in volunteer studies. However, due to its propensity to revert, it was not studied further [59]. A strain of *V. cholerae* 3083, termed Texas Star-SR which produces only the B subunit of cholera toxin, was derived through chemical mutagenesis. While vaccination with this strain afforded good levels of protection against cholera in volunteer studies, about 25 % of vaccinees experienced mild to moderate diarrhea [60].

Production and Characteristics of Current Cholera Vaccine. The current licensed cholera vaccine is composed of inactivated whole cells of *V. cholerae* and is administered parenterally. Fermentor-grown cultures are inactivated by a combination of heat and phenol or formaliin. Usually, two cultures are produced individually to give a combination of Ogawa-classical and Inaba-El Tor serotypes-biotypes and are later mixed in equal amounts. Cell concentration is adjusted to 5-8 x 10^9 cells/dose (0.5 ml). Vaccine potency is estimated by an intraperitoneal mouse challenge test. Two doses of vaccine given at 2-week intervals are recommended. A booster dose is recommended whenever entering an endemic area.

Adverse Reactions. Approximately 20-30 % of vaccinees will have a mild to moderate local reaction consisting of pain, redness, and/or swelling. Systemic reactions such as fever, headache, or malaise occur in ~ 5 % of vaccinees.

Vaccine Efficacy. Various parenteral vaccines, including inactivated whole-cell, purified lipopolysaccharide, cell-free Inaba antigen, and a whole-cell vaccine in adjuvant, have been evaluated in placebo-controlled field trials (for a review see reference [61]). The results from these trials can be summarized as follows: I) two doses of vaccine are superior to 1; II) protection afforded by vaccination is greater in adults than children; III) vaccination is only moderately effective in nonendemic areas; and IV) protection lasts for only 3-6 months. Therefore, the currently available cholera vaccine can not be considered an effective tool to control endemic cholera. It is best employed by travellers entering an endemic area for a short period of time.

Future Prospects. Due to advances in understanding the pathogenesis and molecular genetics of *V. cholerae*, it is likely that one or more safe and effective cholera vaccines will be introduced in the near future.

Several attenuated live oral vaccine strains have been developed by deleting the cholera toxin gene or its enzymatically active A subunit [62, 63]. A derivative of *V. cholerae* 16961, in which the cholera toxin gene was deleted, was found to afford excellent protection (89 %) against clinical disease. However, 50 % of volunteers who ingested the vaccine had mild to moderate diarrhea. A second vaccine strain was produced by deletion of the A subunit of cholera toxin from strain 395. Again, good protection was afforded by a single dose of vaccine, but mild diarrhea was observed in 60 % of subjects after vaccination.

The discovery by O'Brien et al. [64] that strains of *V. cholerae* can produce a Shiga-like cytotoxin suggested that at least part of the diarrhea seen after immunization with the above vaccine strains could be due to this toxin. Therefore, Levine and co-workers [65] deleted the A subunit of cholera toxin from strain 569B which is naturally cytotoxin negative. This strain, called CVD-103, is far less reactogenic than previously evaluated strains, eliciting mild diarrhea in ~ 5 % of North American volunteers, who received a single oral dose of vaccine containing ~ 10^8 bacteria. Vaccination with CVD-103 afforded excellent protection (87 %) against a homologous challenge. Furthermore, significant protection (67-78 %) was seen even when the challenge was of a different serotype or biotype. Protection was found to correlate with a significant rise in serum vibriocidal and antitoxic antibody levels.

The CVD-103 strain has also been evaluated for safety and immunogenicity in adult Thai volunteers. In the initial study, 12 college students who received a single dose of vaccine presented with no adverse reactions and mounted an excellent immune response. A second study was conducted in 200 Thai military recruits, half of whom received CVD-103, while the rest received a placebo consisting of killed *E. coli* K12. Two subjects, who had both received placebo, reported mild diarrhea. However, only about 25 % of the subjects responded with a significant antibody response. This same lot of vaccine elicited an excellent immune response in North American subjects. This finding could not be attributed to either improper storage or administration of the vaccine nor to higher pre-existing antibody titers in the military recruits.

Studies are now in progress to determine if the CVD-103 vaccine can consistently evoke a significant antibody response in non-North American volunteers. The next step would be to determine vaccine safety and immunogenicity in children, who are at high risk for contracting disease of serious consequence in endemic areas.

The O-antigen of *V. cholerae* has been expressed on the surface of *S. typhi* Ty21a by Rowley and co-workers. This vaccine is safe when administered at doses as high as 10^{10} bacteria. Recently, a challenge study was conducted in North American volunteers to determine vaccine efficacy. Three doses of vaccine, each containing 10^{11} viable bacteria, were administered on alternate days. Vaccination stimulated a ≥ 4-fold rise in vibriocidal antibody levels in 36 % of subjects. Immunization afforded only 25 % protection against diarrhea following challenge with *V. cholerae*. However, the stool volume was significantly decreased in the vaccinees as compared to the controls.

Orally administered inactivated vaccines consisting of 1 x 10^{11} killed vibrios and 1 mg of B subunit of cholera toxin or 1 x 10^{11} killed vibrios alone per dose have recently been evaluated in Bangladesh [66]. After 6 months of surveillance, three doses of the combined vaccine afforded 85 % protection against cholera whereas the cells alone were 58 % effective. After 1 year, protection had declined to 62 % for the combined vaccine and 53 % for the cells alone. Studies are now in progress to determine if fewer doses of vaccine afford good protection and the need for the B subunit.

2.8 Vaccines Against Nosocomial Pathogens

The routine usage of broad-spectrum antibiotics, more frequent invasive surgery, an increasing role for immunosuppressive agents in the management of cancer, and the ability to prolong the lives of critically ill patients have led to a dramatic increase of hospital-acquired bacterial infections [67]. It is estimated that in the United States alone nosocomial infections are a contributing factor in ~ 70 000 deaths per year and that the cost of treating such infections exceeds 1 billion dollars [68, 69]. The mortality rate for nosocomial bacteremia and pneumonia, especially when caused by Gram-negative bacilli, has remained unacceptably high (≥ 25 %) even with the introduction of numerous antibacterial agents [68]. Therefore, much effort has been devoted to developing immunological agents for the control of these infections [70].

Etiological Agent and Pathogenesis. Although a vast number of bacterial species have been identified as nosocomial pathogens, *Escherichia coli, Klebsiella* spp., *Pseudomonas aeruginosa,* and *Staphylococcus aureus* account for the majority of serious infections, such as bacteremia and pneumonia [71]. Infection with these agents usually arise due to the translocation of bacteria from the skin, bowel, or nasopharyngeal cavity following disruption of the host's defense systems by trauma, invasive surgical procedures, treatment with antibiotics, or immunosuppressive agents. In most instances, foci of infection are formed from which the bacteria enter the bloodstream. Death when it occurs is most likely attributed to shock.

Production and Characteristics of Currently Available Vaccines. At present, there are no vaccines licensed for use against the four pathogens listed above.

Future Prospects. Attempts to control bacterial nosocomial infections by immunological means are complicated because of the diverse patient populations who are at high risk and the substantial number of bacterial pathogens of varying serotypes involved. Furthermore, vaccination of at-risk patients may not be feasible because of the time needed to mount a protective immune response and because of the fact that a substantial portion of these patients will be unable to mount a significant antibody response. A more effective approach would be to passively immunize patients by using a hyperimmune globulin for intravenous use. Therefore, vaccines developed against nosocomial pathogens would be used to vaccinate healthy donors whose plasma would be processed into such a globulin [72].

Currently, two different approaches are being taken to develop hyperimmune products for use against nosocomial infections. The first is based upon developing vaccines to the relevant serospecific bacterial antigens. The second is to engender an antibody response to a common epitope expressed by the lipopolysaccharide (LPS) of Gram-negative bacteria.

2.8.1 Serospecific Vaccines

1. ***Pseudomonas aeruginosa***

Human immunity to *P. aeruginosa* is dependent upon the presence of humoral antibody directed against serospecific LPS determinants and toxin A [72]. Several LPS-containing vaccines have been developed and clinically evaluated [73]. Although promising results were obtained, these vaccines have not gained wide acceptance due to a combination of toxicity, poor immunogenicity, or poorly characterized antigenic content. Pier and co-workers have purified and tested two serotypes of *P. aeruginosa* high-molecular-weight polysaccharides which were found to be safe and immunogenic in humans [74]. In an attempt to engender both an antitoxin A and an anti-LPS antibody response, toxin A-O-polysaccharide conjugate vaccines have been synthesized. Such conjugates are non-toxic, non-pyrogenic, safe when administered to humans, and evoked an immune response to both vaccine moieties [75]. An octavalent vaccine based upon O-polysaccharide (O-PS) serotypes most frequently causing serious disease has been formulated and evaluated for safety and immunogenicity. This vaccine was found to be well tolerated by healthy adult volunteers and engendered a significant rise in antibody titers to all vaccine components.

2. ***Klebsiella* spp.**

Antibody to *Klebsiella* capsular polysaccharide (CPS) has been shown to be highly protective against experimental infections [76]. Several experimental vaccines composed of purified *Klebsiella* CPS were found to be safe and immunogenic in human volunteers [70]. Based upon the seroepidemiology of *Klebsiella* blood isolates, a 24-valent CPS vaccine has been developed [77]. This vaccine is safe and immunogenic in humans. It also elicits antibodies to 11 "cross-reactive" serotypes of CPS not included in the vaccine and therefore offers potential "coverage" against roughly 75 % of all *Klebsiella* bacteremic isolates. Approximately 100 volunteers have been immunized with the 24-valent vaccine. Reactions have been few and of a mild, transient nature. There is considerable diversity in the magnitude of the immune response elicited among the 24 vaccine antigens themselves and from subject to subject. However, there was a good overall mean antibody response. (≥ 10-fold rise in IgG titer)

3. ***Escherichia coli***

Antibodies to both O (LPS) and K (capsular) antigens can provide significant protection against experimental *E. coli* infections [78, 79]. However, roughly 40 % of *E. coli* bacteremic isolates are non-encapsulated [80]. In addition, the 2 most frequently encountered K serotypes among blood isolates, K1 and K5, are nonimmunogenic in humans due to features shared with mammalian glycosaminoglycans. Approximately 90 % of *E. coli* bacteremic isolates can be typed according to O-antigen. The majority of such isolates can be grouped within 12 serotypes, making a polyvalent formulation feasible [80]. The toxicity of native LPS precludes its use as a vaccine. However, we have found it possible to isolate nontoxic, serologically reactive O-polysaccharide from *E. coli* LPS. Due to their low molecular weight, however, they are nonimmunogenic. We are now in the process of constructing O-PS-protein conjugates in a manner similar to that described for *P. aeruginosa* (see above). Preliminary results indicate *E. coli* O-PS linked to various carrier proteins can induce a protective immune response in animals. A monovalent conjugate vaccine is to be tested in humans for safety and immunogenicity in the near future.

4. *Staphylococcus aureus*

S. aureus produce numerous somatic antigens and extracellular toxins which have been implicated as virulence factors. These include teichoic acid, lipoteichoic acid, exopolysaccharide, capsular polysaccharide, alpha toxin, and β-toxin. Patients with deep-seated *S. aureus* disease usually mount an antibody response to teichoic acid, alpha toxin, and β-toxin [81]. However, the relative protective capacities of antibodies against these antigens are unknown.

Recently, Karakawa and co-workers have described a serotyping scheme for *S. aureus* based upon cell-surface polysaccharide [82]. Approximately 80-90 % of *S. aureus* clinical isolates belong to one of these serotypes, with type 5 and type 8 predominating [83]. Serospecific polysaccharide is produced during experimental *S. aureus* infections and can be isolated from blood [84]. It is possible to purify *S. aureus* CPS [85]. Anti-CPS antibodies can promote the uptake and killing of *S. aureus* by polymorphonuclear leukocytes [86]. Recently, it has been shown that anti-CPS antibody can prevent non-fatal experimental *S. aurus* infections [87]. The safety and immunogenicity of *S. aureus* polysaccharides in humans has not yet been determined.

2.8.2 Cross-reactive Anti-core Glycolipid Vaccine

Antibody engendered against the core glycolipid of *E. coli* strain J5 broadly cross-reacts with the LPS of virtually all Gram-negative bacteria [88]. Polyclonal or monoclonal anti-J5 antibody can afford significant protection against several Gram-negative pathogens [89]. Recent findings indicate that protective antibody is directed against the lipid A moiety of LPS and acts to neutralize the toxic activities of LPS rather than effecting the opsonization of the invading bacteria.

Human plasma enriched for anti-J5 antibody has been found to provide significant protection against death due to "Gram-negative shock" when used prophylactically or therapeutically in non-immunocompromised patients [90, 91]. However, a single dose of human anti-J5 plasma afforded no protection against Gram-negative infections in neutropenic patients [92]. Clinical trials conducted using an intravenous immune globulin (IVIG) obtained from donors immunized with J5 vaccine showed no efficacy as compared to a control group which received normal IVIG [93]. It is important to note that the anti-J5 IVIG possessed ELISA anti-J5 IgG titers of only 2.2-fold higher than the control preparation.

At present, three trials are underway to evaluate additional anti-core glycolipid antibody. One study is evaluating a human anti-J5 IgM monoclonal antibody, while a murine monoclonal antibody is being tested in a second trial. A human polyclonal IVIG preparation obtained from donors immunized with a *Salmonella minnesota* Re mutant is being analyzed in a third trial. Preliminary results indicate that both monoclonal antibodies significantly reduce mortality associated with Gram-negative sepsis.

2.9 Meningococcal Meningitis Vaccine

Etiological Agent and Pathogenesis. The causative agent of meningococcal disease is *Neisseria meningitidis*, a Gram-negative diplococcus. Humans are the only known reservoir for *N. meningitidis*. The meningococcus can colonize the nasopharynx with such asymptomatic carriers often serving to disseminate the disease. Infrequently, the meningococcus enters the bloodstream and infects the meninges. Meningococcal disease is most often seen in children less than 18 months of age and in settings such as military recruit camps where individuals from different geographical areas come into constant close contact [94]. The disease is endemic worldwide with an incidence of about 3/100 000 population per year. There have been numerous epidemics in the past two decades where attack rates exceeding 500/100 000 have been documented. There are 11 known meningococcal capsular serotypes with the majority (~ 95 %) of disease caused by groups A, B, C, W135 and Y [94, 95].

History of Vaccination Against Meningococcal Meningitis. The first attempts at immunizing against meningococcal disease used vaccines made of killed bacteria and were unsuccessful [96]. Attention then centered upon using purified capsular antigens. Kabat demonstrated in 1945 that up to 1 mg of purified antigen could be administered to humans with no untoward reactions. However, these studies were not continued since the prophylactic use of antibiotics appeared to be highly effective at preventing meningococcal meningitis. The appearance of resistant strains of *N. meningitidis* in the early 1960s revived interest in vaccine development. In the late 1960s Gotschlich and co-workers [97] showed that highly purified group A and group C capsular polysaccharides which possessed a high molecular weight were safe and immunogenic in humans. Human immune sera contained elevated levels of antibody capable of mediating the lysis of meningococci in the presence of complement.

Production and Charcteristics of Current Meningococcal Vaccines. Vaccines are available which contain serogroup A, C, W135 and Y capsular antigens. The most widely used formulations are the tetravalent A, C, W135 and Y and the bivalent A and C vaccines. Capsular antigens are purified from fermentor grown cultures by co-precipitation with detergents followed by ethanol fractionation, extraction with organic solvents, and ultracentrifugation. These procedures remove the vast majority of protein, nucleic acids, lipids, and lipopolysaccharide from the capsular antigen. To preserve the high molecular weight of the capsular antigens is of critical importance since this governs the immune response. The vaccines contain 50 μg of capsular antigen per serotype in lyophilized form. Release of the vaccine is based upon various physiochemical properties (size and purity). No animal potency test is required.

Current Recommendations for Vaccine Usage. Meningococcal vaccine can be administered to any immunocompetent individual over 18 months of age. A single dose of vaccine is given either subcutaneously or intramuscularly. The group A antigen is immunogenic in children ≥ 6 months of age, but 2 doses must be administered within a 2-3 month interval. Due to the low incidence of the disease in the general population, vaccine acceptance has been poor. The majority of vaccine is now used to immunize military recruits or travellers.

Adverse Reactions. The meningococcal vaccines are very safe. It is estimated that about 250 000 000 doses of vaccine have been administered worldwide with no vaccine-associated fatalities reported. Mild, transient local reactions occur in about 25 % of vaccinees.

Vaccine Efficacy. Conclusive proof that group C meningococcal vaccine prevents disease was presented by Artenstein et al. in 1970 [98]. Subsequently, the group A vaccine was found to be effective at controlling endemic and epidemic disease in adults and children [99, 100]. Group C vaccine was found to elicit a protective antibody response only in children ≥ 18 months of age, whereas the two doses of group A vaccine were immunogenic in children ≥ 6 months of age [101]. Efficacy for the W135 and Y capsular antigens has not been clinically demonstrated, but is assumed based upon their ability to engender appropriate levels of relevant functional antibodies in humans.

Future Prospects. The current meningococcal vaccines have two major limitations. First, they do not provide protection against group B organisms which can account for up to 50 % of endemic cases in certain areas. Secondly, the group C vaccine is non-immunogenic in children ≤ 18 months of age.

In an attempt to construct meningococcal vaccines capable of engendering a protective immune response in young children, capsular antigens have been coupled to carrier proteins to form conjugate vaccines [102]. Group A and C antigens, when coupled to tetanus toxoid, no longer behave as T-independent antigens, but rather in a T-dependent fashion, at least in animals. Furthermore, the conjugates are more immunogenic than native capsular antigens. Studies are now in progress to determine the safety and immunogenicity of group A and C conjugates in humans.

The major difficulty in producing a group B meningococcal vaccine is that the group B capsular antigen, a homopolymer of α (2→ 8)-linked sialic acid, is poorly immunogenic in humans [103], probably because similar structures are found in human gangliosides and fetal proteins. Even when coupled to carrier proteins [102] or mixed with group B outer membrane proteins [101], the group B antigen is a poor immunogen. An alternative approach is to use serotype-specific outer membrane proteins (OMP). At present, 18 serotypes have been identified based upon OMP. However, serotypes 2 and 15 appear to dominate at present. OMP vaccines containing group B or C capsular antigens have been administered to several thousand humans (adults and children) and were found to be safe and immunogenic [104, 105]. A large scale field trial to determine the efficacy of OMP vaccines is now being conducted. The main problem with the above OMP vaccines is their restricted serospecificity. This has led to the search for common somatic antigens expressed by most invasive group B strains.

2.10 Tuberculosis Vaccine

Etiological Agent and Pathogenesis. Human pulmonary tuberculosis is caused by the acid-fast bacilli, *Mycobacterium tuberculosis* and *M. bovis,* the latter causing disease primarily in children. *M. tuberculosis* is spread by infected droplets, whereas *M. bovis* is disseminated by ingestion of contaminated milk. Currently, the vast majority of clinical disease is among middle-aged individuals in developed countries and in children < 10 years of age in underdeveloped countries. The incidence of tuberculosis presently ranges from 500 per 100 000 population in certain regions of Africa to ~ 10 per 100 000 in Europe and North America. It has been estimated that 95-98 % of people exposed to *M. tuberculosis* subsequently become infected, i.e., become tuberculin positive, but do not manifest signs of clinical disease and are immune to further exposures [106]. Therefore, only a small percentage of infections progress to a disease state. Once the inhaled bacilli reach the lower respiratory tract, they are ingested by alveolar macrophages. Rapid intracelllar growth occurs with inflammatory cell recruitment leading to granuloma formation. In the majority of cases, this is as far as the disease progresses. Active disease can present a variety of clinical symptoms ranging from self-limiting pulmonary involvement to an acute disseminated disease which rapidly leads to death.

History of Vaccination Against Tuberculosis. Efforts to protect humans against tuberculosis have almost exclusively employed BCG (Bacillus Calmette-Guérin) vaccine (see below). BCG vaccine was first evaluated over 60 years ago in newborns who were given three oral doses of vaccine 3, 5 and 7 days after birth. Shortly thereafter, additional studies showed BCG vaccine to be safe when given orally or parenterally. In the early 1930s, Aronson and Overton began large scale trials with BCG vaccine. Subsequent trials involving American Indians and Eskimos showed that intradermally administered BCG conferred protection against disease in infants. Additional proof of vaccine efficacy was obtained in a small scale trial with Canadian Indians [107]. Even in the face of a high disease transmittance rate and a mortality rate of 800/100 000 due to tuberculosis, the vaccine was more than 80 % effective over a 9-year observation period.

Currently Available Tuberculosis Vaccine. The original BCG vaccine strain was developed at the Pasteur Institute over 50 years ago by *in vitro* cultivation of *M. bovis* for 10 years. With the widespread distribution of BCG vaccine, numerous substrains are now used to produce commercial products. The bacteria are grown on Savton's liquid media either in bottles with a high surface area or in submerged culture. The bacteria are collected, suspended in a stabilizer solution, homogenized, and lyophilized. The bulk material is standardized by opacity, dry weight and number of viable bacteria per unit weight. The vaccine is usually filled into glass ampules which are sealed under vacuum.

Controls of BCG vaccine are stringent. First, the culture is examined for purity, viability, and identity. Innocuousness is tested by injection of vaccine into guinea pigs. The number of live organisms are determined by viability counting. General safety tests to document absence of unexpected toxicity are also performed. Resistance of the bacteria to elevated temperatures is also documented. Currently, vaccine potency is based upon the total viable bacteria per dose. However, this is not totally satisfactory for the following reasons: I) different strains of BCG may vary in their ability to evoke a protective cell-mediated immune (CMI) response; and II) the ratio of viable to non-viable bacteria can influence the magnitude of both the humoral and CMI response to vaccination [108].

Current Recommendations for Vaccine Usage. A single intradermal dose containing 4-8 x 10^5 viable organisms in 0.1 ml is normally administered. Depending upon the circumstances, BCG vaccine can be administered to immunocompetent infants or adults with good results. The preferred use of BCG vaccine depends upon the disease incidence in the area in question. In developed areas, such as Europe or North America where disease is infrequent, vaccination should be limited to individuals at high risk to exposure including family members of tuberculosis patients, health care workers expected to come into contact with tuberculosis patients or infected clinical specimens, and travellers entering an area of high endemicity for a prolonged period of time. In developing areas with a high rate of disease incidence, routine immunization of infants is felt to be a cost-effective method of controlling tuberculosis. In addition, all tuberculin-negative children upon entry into schools and tuberculin-negative adults should be vaccinated.

Adverse Reactions to Vaccination With BCG. BCG vaccine, when administered properly in the correct dosage, is considered to be a safe vaccine. A report by Lotte and co-workers [109] estimates that 1 vaccination per 100 000 will result in a noticeable reaction. A significant proportion of such reactions are ulcers caused by inadvertently administering the vaccine subcutaneously. Of greater concern are the reports of mycobacterial disease following immunization [110]. Great care must be taken to insure that a potential vaccinee is not immunocompromised as the vaccine organisms can then rapidly multiply and lead to death [111].

Vaccine Efficacy. Numerous controlled field trials, most involving infants or children, have been conducted to evaluate the efficacy of BCG vaccine. Efficacy ranged from 0 % to 80 % (for a review, see reference [106]). Although the three most recent BCG trials failed to document significant vaccine-induced protection and the currently available lyophylized vaccine formulation was found to afford no protection in a South Indian field trial, there continues to be considerable support for large scale vaccination in developing countries [112].

Future Prospects. At present, there are no "second-generation" tuberculosis vaccines being clinically evaluated. Although the tuberculin skin test offers a practical method to measure "immunity" to disease, we do not know precisely what induces a tuberculin-positive state at the molecular level. Ideally, a new vaccine would be comprised of either purified *M. tuberculosis* protective antigens or the appropriate antigens expressed by a live-attenuated carrier.

Recently, several *M. tuberculosis* cell surface antigens have been identified which can induce a CMI response in experimental animals [113]. The cloning of such antigens and their high-level expression in bacteria or yeast would allow for economical large scale purification. Alternatively, such cloned genes could be inserted into a vector such as vaccinia virus which has been shown to be an excellent vehicle for numerous other recombinant proteins [114]. Given the fact that most tuberculosis vaccine will be used in underdeveloped nations, any new vaccine must not only be safe and effective, but also economical to produce and control.

2.11 *Escherichia coli* Vaccines

Etiological Agent and Pathogenesis. *Escherichia coli* , a Gram-negative motile rod, is a leading cause of diarrheal disease, urinary tract infections, neonatal meningitis, and nosocomial infections. *E. coli* produces a variety of virulence factors including a polysaccharide capsule (K antigen), lipopolysaccharide (LPS; O-antigen), fimbriae, enterotoxins, and cytotoxins. The relative importance of these factors depends upon the anatomical site of the infection. In addition, the majority of *E. coli* strains causing a given disease fall within a limited number of K or O serotypes.

E. coli is the leading cause of diarrhea worldwide. Three "categories" of *E. coli* strains are recognized based upon the disease syndrome they cause. Enterotoxigenic *E. coli* (ETEC) invariably causes watery diarrhea which can be accompanied by cramps, fever, or vomiting. The disease is acquired by ingesting contaminated foodstuffs and affects infants, young children, and travellers to underdeveloped countries. ETEC strains produce either a heat-stable enterotoxin (ST), a heat-labile enterotoxin (LT), or both. ETEC strains also possess fimbriae which mediate attachment to the ileal epithelium. Three distinct fimbriae, termed CFA/I, CFA/II and E8775, have been identified on ETEC strains isolated from human disease. Once colonization of the small bowel is accomplished, the action of ST and/or LT results in the disease symptoms noted.

Enteroinvasive *E. coli* (EIEC) cause a dysentery-like disease characterized by fever, diarrhea, cramps, and stools containing blood and mucous. IEEC is acquired by ingestion of contaminated food. EIEC disease occurs with approximately equal frequency worldwide. EIEC can readily penetrate the ileal and colonic epithelium where the bacteria undergo rapid multiplication resulting in tissue destruction. EIEC can then infect adjacent cells or penetrate to the lamina propria.

Enteropathogenic *E. coli* (EPEC) affect primarily infants and young children after ingestion of contaminated food causing watery diarrhea often accompanied by fever and/or vomiting. EPEC strains rarely produce ST or LT, nor are they able to invade eucaryotic cells. EPEC strains colonize the ileal epithelium with marked destruction of the surrounding brush-border in the absence of invasion. EPEC strains can elaborate a cytotoxin similar to that produced by *Shigella dysenteriae* 1 which is called Shiga-like toxin. It is believed the action of Shiga-like toxin elicits the clinical symptoms.

Approximately 50 % of neonatal meningitis is due to *E. coli.* Transmission of the infecting strain is from mother to infant. It appears that *E. coli* penetrates the intestinal epithelium of the neonate and enters the bloodstream from which it is translocated to the meninges. The majority of strains (> 80 %) causing meningitis express the K1 capsular antigen. However, O-antigen type in addition to the K1 phenotype appear to play a role in virulence. *E. coli* meningitis carries a high attendant fatality rate.

E. coli is the causative agent of approximately 90 % of non-obstructive urinary tract infections (UTI). The clinical syndromes can include bacteriuria, cystitis and pyelonephritis.

UTI's are much more common among women than men. Renal scarring associated with pyelonephritis occurs most often in children ≤5 years of age. The infecting organisms are thought to be acquired from the flora colonizing the vagina and periurethral areas. P and type 1 fimbriae are believed to play an important role in UTI's by mediating tissue colonization [115].

History of Immunization Against *E. coli* Disease. Initial attempts to vaccinate against *E. coli* diarrhea used crude Boivin extracts derived from 0 types 111, 55 and 86 [116]. In one study, infants (birth - 1 year of age) who were hospitalized received multiple doses of orally administered vaccine. Overall efficacy was 41 %.

Studies conducted by Levine et al. [117]. demonstrated that volunteers fed an LT/ST positive strain of *E. coli* who responded with diarrhea were protected upon subsequent challenge with the homologous strain. Surprisingly, the number of *E. coli* shed in the feces of control and "immunized" subjects was comparable. This was taken to indicate that protection was mediated by toxin-neutralizing and/or colonization-inhibiting rather than bactericidal antibody. Based upon these pioneering studies, efforts to develop vaccines against *E. coli* diarrhea have focused upon inducing antitoxic or anti-attachment antibody.

To address the relative protective capacity of antitoxic immunity, Levine et al. [117] challenged volunteers who recovered from diarrhea due to an LT/ST positive strain with an LT-only strain of *E. coli* differing in O and H serotypes. No protection was observed indicating that anti-LT immunity is of itself insufficient to afford protection. Similar results were obtained when volunteers who were immunized with the *V. cholerae* CVD-103 HgR vaccine strain discussed above were challenged with an LT/ST positive strain (M.M. Levine, personal communication).

Attempts to protect against *E. coli* diarrhea based upon the induction of anti-colonization factor antibody have shown more promise. Graded doses (45-1800 μg) of purified type I fimbriae have been parenterally administered to human volunteers [118]. The vaccine was well tolerated and elicited both a humoral IgG and an intestinal secretory IgA antibody response. Six volunteers who received a primary vaccine dose of 45 or 90 μg and a booster dose of 1800 μg on day 28 were challenged with an ST^+, LT^+, CFA^+, Type I $pili^+$strain of *E. coli*. Two of the six vaccinees became ill compared with seven of the seven controls. Additional studies showed that protection was not significant when lower immunizing doses were used and that protection was seen only when the challenge strain possessed fimbriae homologous to the vaccine [118]. Oral administration of 1 mg of purified CFA/I evoked a significant secretory IgA response in about 50 % of human vaccinees [119]. Responders were protected against challenge with an ST^+, LT^+, CFA/I^+ *E coli* strain.

Rowe et al. (see in [120]) have described the isolation of a spontaneous mutant of *E. coli* strain E1392-75-2A which has lost the genes for ST and LT production, but still expresses CFA/II. When graded doses of this strain were fed to volunteers, a moderate serum IgG antibody response to LPS and CFA/II was induced. However, 2 of 15 volunteers who received $\geq 10^{10}$ organisms experienced mild diarrhea.

Currently Available Vaccines Against *E. coli* Infections. There are currently no vaccines available to prevent *E. coli* diarrhea, UTI's, or meningitis.

Future Prospects. At present, both attenuated live-oral and inactivated vaccines are being evaluated as to their ability to prevent *E. coli* diarrhea. Recently, Evans et al. [119] have described the production of a killed inactivated, orally-administered whole cell vaccine (strain H-10407; ST^+, LT^+, 0,78, H11, CFA/I^+). The majority of vaccinees responded with a good secretory IgA antibody response to CFA/I. The diarrhea attack rate for volunteers challenged with a toxicogenic CFA/I$^+$ *E. coli* strain was 89 % for those in the placebo group and 20 % for those in the vaccine group.

There is considerable interest in using live-attenuated carrier strains, such as *E. coli* E1392-75-2A or *S. typhi* Ty21a [50] to deliver critical protective antigens such as colonization factors or enterotoxoids [120]. Prototype strains are now being constructed and will hopefully be available for clinical evaluation in the near future. Several purified antigen preparations also hold promise as *E. coli* diarrhea vaccine candidates. These include ST-LT conjugates [121], the B subunit of LT [122], and an LT toxoid termed "procoligenoid" produced by the controlled heating of LT [123].

Since the majority of *E. coli* strains associated with neonatal meningitis possess the K1 capsule, this would appear to be an excellent vaccine candidate. However, the K1 antigen which is identical to the group B meningococcal capsule is not immunogenic in humans. Several group B meningococcal vaccines have been developed and some are undergoing clinical evaluation (see section on meningococcal meningitis). If one of these vaccines can induce good levels of functional IgG antibody (which is able to cross the placenta), it could be used to vaccinate pregnant women.

At present the most promising vaccines to prevent serious *E. coli* UTI's, i.e., pyelonephritis, contain type I fimbrial antigens. Schmidt et al. [124] have identified 2 fimbrial amino acid sequences which prevent colonization by a homologous strain in a murine pyelonephritis model. In addition, antibody to one sequence was also capable of affording protection against a strain of *E. coli* expressing a distinct fimbrial serotype.

2.12 *Neisseria gonorrhoeae* Vaccine

Etiological Agent and Pathogenesis. *Neisseria gonorrhoeae* was identified as the causative agent of gonorrhea by Bumm in 1885. It is a Gram-negative dipplococcus with humans serving as its only known natural host. Gonorrhea is a sexually transmitted disease of epidemic proportions worldwide. More than 500 000 cases are reported annually in the United States. In most instances, the infection remains restricted to its entry site, i.e., the genitalia, pharynx, and/or rectum. The majority (> 90 %) of infected males display symptoms characterized by pain upon urination and an urethral exudate [125]. However, up to 50 % of infected women remain asymptomatic and can serve as carriers. In approximately 10 % of women with genital gonorrhea, the bacteria invades the bloodstream and results in pelvic inflammatory disease. Disseminated gonococcal infections are far less frequent in male patients.

When cultured on solid medium, 4 colonial variants, called T1-T4, can be discerned [126]. Of critical importance is the fact that only T1 and T2 variants, which are piliated, can cause disease [127]. The first step in the infectious process is pili-mediated attachment of the gonococcus to mucus-secreting epithelial cells. Shortly thereafter, the bacteria are internalized and translocate to the submucous area. This process can lead to localized alteration of the epithelial surface. Various outer membrane proteins, lipopolysaccharide and proteolytic enzymes may play a role in this process [125]. Treatment of gonorrhea has recently been complicated by the occurrence of multiply resistant clinical isolates.

History of Vaccination Against Gonorrhea. The first attempt to prevent gonorrhea by immunization used a killed whole cell vaccine administered parenterally [128]. This vaccine afforded no protection against the disease in Eskimos. Subsequent human vaccine trials have centered around the use of purified intact pili. Anti-pili antibody is known to block attachment of the gonococcus to epithelial cells. In addition, an anti-pili secretory IgA antibody response is mounted during natural infection [129]. Purified *N. gonorrhoeae* pili were found to be safe upon parenteral administration to volunteers [129]. Vaccination elicited a humoral and a local vaginal antibody response. These antibodies were able to block the attachment of *N. gonorrhoeae* to epithelial cells *in vitro* [129]. Two 2 mg doses of a monovalent pili vaccine resulted in significant protection against challenge with the homologous strain [130]. However, no protection was observed when the challenge strain possessed a pilus serotype modestly cross-reactive with the vaccine [125]. A subsequent field trial with this monovalent vaccine failed to show any protection among military personnel in Korea [129].

Currently Available Gonorrhea Vaccines. At present, no vaccine has been licensed for the prevention of gonorrhea.

Future Prospects. The above human volunteers studies have shown that protection against gonorrhea mediated by anti-pili antibody is serospecific [129]. Two different approaches are now being taken to circumvent the problem of antigenic variation among pili of different isolates. A polyvalent vaccine containing those types of pili which predominate in a given area has been proposed [139]. The two drawbacks to this approach are the large quantities of antigen needed for such a vaccine (~ 1 mg of pili per type) and the distinct possibility that vaccination will create positive selective pressure for the emergence of nonvaccine pili types.

Perhaps a more promising approach would be to utilize conserved antigenic domains with the pili molecule. Schoolnik et al. [131] have identified a cyanogen bromide cleavage fragment which induces antibody able to recognize various pili types. Peptides corresponding to this conserved region have been shown to block attachment of the gonococcus to epithelial cells *in vitro* [132]. If such peptides can induce a broadly protective immune response in humans, it would be feasible to couple synthetic peptides containing the proper sequence onto carrier proteins to produce a conjugate vaccine.

A possible alternative to pili as vaccine antigens are the outer membrane proteins of *N. gonorrhoeae*. The most promising candidate at this time appears to be the PI protein. PI protein has a sufficiently restricted antigenic variation to make construction of a polyvalent vaccine feasible. Furthermore, anti-PI antibody is bactericidal and may block entry of the gonococcus into epithelial cells [133]. An outer membrane preparation enriched for PI protein has been shown to be safe when parenterally administered to humans and to elicit an antibody response [134]. Challenge studies are now being conducted to determine if immunization with PI protein can afford protection against disease.

2.13 *Haemophilus influenzae* Type B Vaccines

Etiological Agent and Pathogenesis. *Haemophilus influenzae* is a Gram-negative bacillus first isolated by Pfeiffer in 1892. The vast majority (> 90 %) of human disease is caused by type B capsular serotype organisms. Most *H. influenzae* type B disease occurs in children between the ages of 3 months to 2 years and corresponds to a time when bactericidal antibody levels are extremely low [135]. *H. influenzae* type B can be the cause of several serious disease syndromes predominated by meningitis. *H. influenzae* type B meningitis is endemic worldwide and constitutes one of the three leading causes of bacterial meningitis in developed countries. Infection is by inhalation of contaminated aerosols. After localized multiplication, the organisms enter into the bloodstream and translocate to the meninges. Even though effective antibiotic treatment regimens against *H. influenzae* type B have been available for many years, meningitis due to this organism still has a high attendant morbidity and mortality rate.

History of Immunization Against *H. influenzae* Type B Disease. Intensive efforts to understand how human immunity to *H. influenzae* type B disease is mediated has, for the most part, replaced clinical trials which use crude, poorly characterized vaccines. The capsular polysaccharide is a critical virulence factor of *H. influenzae* type B conferring resistance to lysis in serum [136]. It is now known that antibody-dependent, complement-mediated bacteriolysis is the basis for immunity against *H. influenzae* type B [136]. Antibodies directed against the type B capsular polysaccharide are known to be bactericidal in the presence of complement and are believed to be the predominant protective antibody [135]. Therefore, vaccine development has centered around the use of purified type B capsular polysaccharide.

Production and Characteristics of Current *H. influenzae* Type B Vaccines. There are now two vaccines licensed for use against *H. influenzae* type B, a purified capsular polysaccharide and a conjugate vaccine composed of capsular polysaccharide covalently coupled to diphtheria toxoid. Production of both vaccines centers around the purification of the capsular antigen. This is accomplished by co-precipitation of the capsule with detergent, digestion with nucleases and proteases, extraction in phenol, and ultracentrifugation. For the construction of the conjugate vaccine, the polysaccharide is covalently linked to diphtheria toxoid by a bifunctional spacer molecule. There is no animal potency test for *H. influenzae* type B vaccines. Rather, release, i.e. potency, is determined by analysis of various physiochemical characteristics which serve to identify and quantitate the capsular antigen and confirm that it is an immunogenic form.

Current Immunization Recommendations. The capsular polysaccharide vaccine was first licensed for use in the United States in 1985. At present, a single 25 μg dose, administered parenterally, is recommended for children 2-6 years of age. No booster dose is needed. For the conjugate vaccine licensed in December 1987, a single dose is recommended for children 18 months-6 years of age. No booster dose is needed.

Vaccine Efficacy. The purified capsular polysaccharide vaccine was evaluated in a placebo-controlled trial among 100 000 Finnish children 3 months to 5 years of age [137]. Vaccine efficacy was approximately 90 % for children who were vaccinated at 24 months of age or older over a 2-year period of observation. Vaccination provided no protection in children 18 months of age or younger due to poor immunogenicity {137]. Efficacy was found to correlate with anti-capsular polysaccharide titers of > 0.15 μg/ml. Immunization of 18-month-old children elicited protective antibody levels in only 50 % of the vaccinees [138].

Recently, considerable controversy has surrounded the use of this vaccine due to lower than expected efficacy based upon post-marketing case-control studies (see reference [139] for summary). Point efficacy estimates ranged from -86 % to 89 %. The consensus is that overall protection is about 50-60 %. This relatively poor showing has been attributed in great part to the poor immunogenicity of the vaccine, especially among certain minority populations which may have a genetic disposition to respond poorly to polysaccharide vaccines [140, 141].

The diphtheria toxoid-capsular polysaccharide conjugate vaccine was licensed for use in 18 month-old children based upon its ability to evoke protective levels of antibodies [142]. This vaccine has, in effect, replaced the capsular polysaccharide vaccine. Post-marketing efficacy studies for this vaccine have not yet been published.

Future Prospects. A *H. influenzae* type B vaccine is clearly needed in young children (≤ 18 months of age). Such a vaccine should be compatible with current infant immunization programs using combined diphtheria, tetanus, and pertussis vaccine, e.g., a quadrivalent vaccine. Several vaccine candidates exist including the diphtheria toxoid conjugate discussed above, a conjugate formed by covalently coupling the polysaccharide to either CRM 197 (a nontoxic mutant diphtheria "toxoid") [143] or tetanus toxoid [144], and a non-covalently coupled vaccine prepared by combining the polysaccharide with *N. meningitidis* group B outer membrane protein [145]. These vaccines are currently undergoing clinical evaluation for safety, immunogenicity, and efficacy in 3-6 month-old infants.

Efficacy data are currently available only for the diphtheria toxoid conjugate vaccine. In a Finnish study, the vaccine was administered to infants at 3, 4, 6 and 14 months of age. After 5 months of surveillance, efficacy was 83 % in children who received 3 doses of vaccine, which induced a significant rise in antibody titers [146]. Continued follow-up (~ 15 months) gave the following point efficacy estimates: for children who received 1 or 2 doses, 66 %; for 3 doses, 87 %; and for 4 doses, 100 %.

Another study was conducted with this vaccine in which native Alaskan (Eskimo) children received the vaccine at 2, 4, and 6 months of age [147]. Point efficacy studies were 25 % following the first dose, 0 % after 2 doses, and 39 % after 3 doses. This degree of protection was not significant and was associated with a very poor antibody response (geometric mean titer of 200 ng/ml) for 9 month-old children.

The precise reasons for the discrepancies between these trials have not yet been identified, but may be due to one or more of the following: I) a difference in genetic background which modulates the immune response; II) interference by maternal antibodies when the initial vaccine dose was given at 2 months compared to 3 months of age; and/or III) lower age of disease incidence in the Alaskan versus the Finnish trial site.

2.14 References

1. Collier, R. J., *Bacteriol. Rev.* (1975), **39**, 54-85.
2. Pappenheimer, A. M., Jr., *In:* Bacterial Vaccines. Germanier, R. (ed.), Academic Press, Orlando, FL, (1984), 1-36.
3. Audibert, F., Jolivet, M., Chedid, L., Alouf, J. E., Boquet, P., Rivaille, P. and Siffert, O., *Nature* (1981), **289**, 593-594.
4. Uchida, T., Gill, D. M. and Pappenheimer, A. M., Jr., *Nature* (1971), **283**, 8-11.
5. Greenfield, L., Dovey, H. L., Lawyer, F. C. and Gelfand, D. H., *Biotechnol.* (1986), **4**, 1006-1011.
6. Bizzini, B., *In:* Bacterial Vaccines. Germanier, R. (ed.), Academic Press, Orlando, FL, (1984), 37-68.
7. Hardegree, M. C., Fornwald, R. E., Farber, J., London, W. T., Parks, F., Kessler, M. J. and Rastogi, S. C., *Proc. Int. Conf. Tetanus* (1982), **6th, 1981**, 409-423.
8. Huet, M., *Proc. Int. Conf. Tetanus* (1982), **6th, 1981**, 425-433.
9. Newell, K. W., Dueñas-Lehmann, A., Leblanc, D. R. and Garces-Osorio, N., *Bull. WHO* (1966), **35**, 863-871.
10. Guerin, N. and Fillastre, C., *Proc. Int. Conf. Tetanus* (1982), **6th, 1981**, 477-479.
11. Pittman, M., *Rev. Infect. Dis.* (1979), **1**, 401-412.
12. Manclark, C. R. and Cowell, J. L., *In:* Bacterial Vaccines, Germanier, R. (ed.), Academic Press, Orlando, FL, (1984), 69-106.
13. Madsen, T., *J. Am. Med. Assoc.* (1933), **101**, 187-188.
14. Cody, C. L., Baraff, L. F., Cherry, J. D., Marcy, S. M.and Manclark, C. R., *Pediatrics* (1981), **68**, 650-660.
15. Aldersdale, R., Bellman, M. H., Rawson, N. S. B., Ross, E. M. and Miller, D. L., *In:* Whooping Cough. Reports from the Committee on Safety of Medicines and the Joint Committee on Vaccination and Immunization. **Vol. IV**, H.M. Stationary Office, London, England, (1981), 79-169.
16. Oda, M., Colwell, J. L., Burstyn, D. G. and Manclark, C. R., *J. Infect. Dis.* (1984), **150**, 823-833.
17. Ad Hoc Group for the Study of Pertussis Vaccines, *Lancet* (1988), **i**, 955-960.
18. Kimura, M. and Kuno-Sakai, H., *Lancet* (1988), **i**, 881-882.
19. Anonymous, *Lancet* (1989), **i**, 114.
20. Chuttani, C. S., Prakash, K., Gupta, P., Grover, V. and Kumar, A., *Bull. WHO* (1977), **55**, 643-644.
21. Reiman, M., *J. Infect. Dis.* (1967), **117**, 101-107.
22. Germanier, R. and Fürer, E., *J. Infect. Dis.* (1975), **131**, 553-558.
23. Gilman, R. H., Hornick, R. B., Woodward, W. E., Dupont, H. L., Snyder, M. J., Levine, M. M. and Libonati, J. P., *J. Infect. Dis.* (1977), **136**, 717-723.
24. Wahdan, M. H., Sérié, C., Cerisier, Y., Sallam, S. and Germanier, R., *J. Infect. Dis.* (1982), **145**, 292-295.
25. World Health Organization Committee on Biological Standardization, *World Health Organization Technical Report,* **series 700**, Geneva, Switzerland (1984), **34th report**, 48-68.
26. Germanier, R., *In:* Bacterial Vaccines, Germanier, R. (ed.), Academic Press, Orlando, FL, (1984), 137-165.
27. Levine, M. M., Ferreccio, C, Black, R. E., Germanier, R. and Chilean Typhoid Committee, *Lancet* (1987), **ii**, 1049-1052.
28. Cryz, S. J., Jr., Fürer, E. and Levine, M. M., *Schweiz. Med. Wschr.* (1988), **118**, 467-470.
29. Simanjuntak, C. H., Paleologo, F. P., Punjabi, N. H., Darmowigoto, R., Soeprawato and Hoffman, S. L., *Abstr. Intersci. Conf. Antimicrob. Agents Chemother* (1988), **28th, 1988**, 308.
30. Levine, M. M., Herrington, D., Murphy, J. R., Morris, J. G., Losonsky, G., Tall, B., Lindberg, A. A., Svenson, S., Baquar, S., Edwards, M. F. and Stocker, B., *J. Clin. Invest.* (1987), **79**, 888-902.
31. Tacket, C., Ferreccio, E., Robbins, J. B., Tsai, C.-M., Schuldz, D., Cadoz, M., Groudeau, A., Levine, M. M., *J. Infect. Dis.* (1986), **154**, 342-345.

32. Acharya, I. L., Lowe, C. V., Thapa, R., Gurubacharya, V., Shrestha, M. B., Cadoz, M., Schultz, D., Armand, J., Bryla, D., Trollfors, B., Campton, T., Schneerson, R. and Robbins, J. B., *N. Engl. J. Med.* (1987), **317**, 1101-1104.
33. Klugman, K. P., Gilbertson, I. T., Koornhof, H. J., Robbins, J. B., Schneerson, R., Schulz, D., Cadoz, M. and Armand, R., *Lancet* (1987), **ii**, 1165-1169.
34. Austrian, R., *Trans. Am. Clin. Climatol. Assoc.* (1977), **89**, 141-161.
35. MacLeod, C. M. and Krauss, M. R., *J. Exp. Med.* (1947), **86**, 439-453.
36. Robbins, J. B., Austrian, R., Lee, C.-J., Rastogi, S. C., Schiffman, G., Henrichsen, J., Mäkelä, P. H., Broome, C. V., Racklam, R. R., Tiesjema, R. H. and Parke, J. C., Jr., *J. Infect. Dis.* (1983), **148**, 1136-1159.
37. Health and Public Policy Committee, American College of Physicians, (1986), **104**, 118-120.
38. Smit, P., Oberholzer, D., Hayden-Smith, S., Koornhof, H. J., et al., *J. Am. Med. Assoc.* (1977), **238**, 2613-2616.
39. Bolan, G., Broome, C. V., Facklam, R. R., Plikaytis, B. D., Fraser, D. W. and Schlech, W. F., *Annals Intern. Med.* (1986), **104**, 1-6.
40. Simberkoff, M. S., Cross, A. P., Al-Ibrahim, M., Baltch, A. L., Geisller, P. J., Nadler, J., Richmond, A. S., Smith, R. P., Schiffman, G., Shepard, D. S. and van Eeckhaut, J. P., *N. Engl. J. Med.* (1986), **315**, 1318-1327.
41. Leech, J. A., Gervais, A. and Ruben, F. L., *Can. Med. Assoc. J.*, (1987), **136**, 361-365.
42. Chu, C., Schneerson, R., Robbins, J. B. and Rastogi, S. C., *Infect. Immun.* (1983), **40**, 245-256.
43. Schneerson, R., Robbins, J. R., Chu, C., Sutton, A., Vann, W., Vickers, J. C., London, W. T., Curman, B., Hardegree, M. C., Shiloach, J. and Rastogi, S. C., *Infect. Immun.* (1984), **45**, 582-591.
44. Schneerson, R., Robbins, J. B., Parke, J. C. Jr., Bell, C., Schlesselman, J. C., Sutton, A., Wang, Z., Schiffman, G., Karpas, A. and Shiloach, J., *Infect. Immun.* (1986), **52**, 519-528.
45. O'Brien, A. D., Thompson, M. R., Gemski, P., Doctor, B. P. and Formal, S. B., *Infect Immun.* (1977), **15**, 796-798.
46. Higgins, A. R., Floyd, T. M. and Kader, M. A., *Am. J. Trop. Med. Hyg.* (1955), **4**, 281-288.
47. Mel, D. M., Gangarosa, E. J., Radovanovic', M. L., Arsic', B. L. and Litvinjenko, S., *Bull. WHO* (1971), **45**, 457-464.
48. Levine, M. M., Rice, P. A., Gangarosa, E. J., Morris, G. K., Snyder, M. J., Formal, S. B., Wells, J. G., Gemski, P., Jr. and Hammond, J., *Am. J. Epidemiol.* (1973), **99**, 30-36.
49. Formal, S. B. and Levine, M. M., *In:* Bacterial Vaccines, Germanier, R. (ed.), Academic Press, Orlando, FL, (1984), p. 167-186.
50. Formal, S. B., Baron, L. S., Kopecko, D. J., Washington, O., Powell, C. and Life, C. A., *Infect. Immun.* (1981), **34**, 746-750.
51. Black, R. E., Levine, M. M., Clements, M. L., Losonsky, G., Herrington, D., Berman, S. and Formal, S. B., *J. Infect. Dis.* (1987), **155**, 1260-1265.
52. Seid, R. C., Jr., Kopecko, D. J., Sadoff, J. C. and Schneider, H., *J. Biolog. Chem.* (1984), **259**, 9028-9034.
53. Baron, L. S., Kopecko, D. J., Formal, S. B., Seid, R., Guerry, P. and Powell, C., *Infect. Immun.* (1987), **55**, 2797-2801.
54. Sturm, S. and Timmis, K., *Microbiol. Pathogenesis* (1986), **1986**, 289-297.
55. Finkelstein, R. A., *Immunol.* (1975), **69**, 137-195.
56. Freter, R. and Gangarosa, E. J., *J. Immunol.* (1961), **91**, 724-730.
57. Cash, R. A., Music, S. I., Libonati, J. P., Craig, J. P., Pierce, N. F. and Hornick, R. B., *J. Infect. Dis.* (1974), **130**, 325-333.
58. Cash, R. A., Music, S. I., Libonati, J. P., Schwartz, A. R. and Hornick, R. B., *Infect. Immun.* (1974), **10**, 762-764.
59. Woodward, W. E., Gilman, R. H., Hornick, R. B., Libonati, J. P. and Cash, R. A., *Dev. Biol. Stand.* (1976), **33**, 108-112.
60. Levine, M. M., Black, R. E., Clements, M. L., Lanata, C., Sears, S., Honda, T., Young, C. R. and Finkelstein, R. A., *Infect. Immun.* (1984), **43**, 515-522.
61. Finkelstein, R. A., *CRC Crit. Rev.* (1973), **2**, 553-623.

62. Kaper, J. B. and Levine, M. M., *Lancet* (1981), **ii**, 1162-1163.
63. Mekalanos, J. J., Suartz, D. J., Pearson, G. D. N., Harford, N., Groyne, F. and de Wilde, M., *Nature* (1983), **306**, 551-557.
64. O'Brien, A. D., Chen, M. E., Holmes, R. K., Kaper, J. and Levine, M. M., *Lancet* (1984), **ii**, 77-78.
65. Levine, M. M., Kaper, J. B., Herrington, D., Ketley, J., Losonsky, G., Tacket, C. O., Tall, B. and Cryz, S., *Lancet* (1988), **ii**, 467-470.
66. Clements, J. D., Harris, J. R., Khan, M. R., Kay, B. A., Yunus, M., Svennerholm, A.-M., Sock, D. A., Chakrabarty, J., Stanton, B. F., Khan, M. V., Atkinson, W. and Holmgren, J., *Lancet* (1986), **ii**, 124-127.
67. McGowan, J. E., Barnes, M. W. and Finland, M., *J. Infect. Dis.* (1975), **132**, 316-335.
68. Bryan, C. S., Reynolds, K. L. and Brenner, E. R., *Rev. Infect. Dis.* (1983), **5**, 629-638.
69. Haley, R. W., *Proc. Internat. Workshop, Baiersbronn, Germany* (1977), 93-95.
70. Cryz, S. J., Jr., *Vaccine* (1987), **5**, 261-265.
71. Jarvis, W. R., White, J. W., Munn, V. P., Mosser, J. L., Emori, T. G., Culver, D. H., Thornsberry, C. and Hughes, J. M., *Centers for Disease Control Surveillance Summaries* (1985), **33, No. 229**, 955-2155.
72. Pollack, M. S. and Young, L. S., *J. Clin. Invest.* (1979), **63**, 276-286.
73. Cryz, S. J., Jr., *In:* Bacterial Vaccines, Germanier, R. (ed.), Academic Press, Orlando, FL, (1984), 317-351.
74. Pier, G. B. and Bennett, S. E., *J. Clin. Invest.* (1986), **77**, 491-495.
75. Cryz, S. J., Jr., Fürer, E., Cross, A. S., Wegmann, A., Germanier, R. and Sadoff, J. C., *J. Clin. Invest.* (1987), **80**, 51-56.
76. Cryz, S. J., Jr., Cross, A. S., Fürer, E., Chariatte, N., Sadoff, J. C. and Germanier, R., *J. Lab. Clin. Med.* (1986), **108**, 182-189.
77. Granström, M., Wertlind, B., Marrman, B. and Cryz, S. J., Jr., *J. Clin. Microbiol.* (1988), **26**, 2257-2261.
78. Welch, W. D., Martin, W. J., Stevens, P. and Young, L. S., *Scand. J. Infect. Dis.* (1979), **11**, 291-298.
79. Kaijser, B. and Ahlstedt, S., *Infect. Immun.* (1977), **17**, 286-289.
80. Cross, A. S., Gemski, P., Sadoff, J. C., Ørskov, F. and Ørskov, I., *J. Infect. Dis.* (1984), **149**, 184-193.
81. Granström, M., Julander, I. and Möllby, R., *Scand. J. Infect. Dis.* (Suppl.) (1983), **41**, 132-139.
82. Karakawa, W. W., Fournier, J. M., Vann, W. F., Arbeit, R., Schneerson, R. S. and Robbins, J. B., *J. Clin. Microbiol.* (1985), **22**, 445-447.
83. Hochkeppel, H. K., Braun, D. G., Visher, W., Imm, A., Sutter, S., Staeuble, V., Guggenheim, R., Kaplan, E. L., Boutonnier, A. and Fournier, J. M., *J. Clin. Microbiol.* (1987), **25**, 526-530.
84. Arbeit, R. D. and Nelles, J. M., *J. Infect. Dis.* (1987), **155**, 242-246.
85. Fournier, J.-M., Vann, W. F. and Karakawa, W., *Infect. Immun.* (1984), **45**, 87-93.
86. Karakawa, W. W., Sutton, A., Schneerson, R., Karpos, A. and Vann, W. F., *Infect. Immun.* (1988), **56**, 1090-1095.
87. Lee, J.C., Perez, N. E., Hopkins, C. A. and Pier, G. B., *J. Infect. Dis.* (1988), **157**, 723-730.
88. Muthoria, L. M., Crockford, G., Bogard, W. C., Jr., and Hancock R. E. W., *Infect. Immun.* (1984), **45**, 723-730.
89. Ziegler, E. J., McCutchan, J. A., Douglas, H. and Braude, A. I., *J. Immunol.* (1973), **111**, 433-438.
90. Ziegler, E. J., McCutchan, J. A., Fierer, J., Glauser, M. P., Sadoff, J. C., Douglas, H. and Braude, A. I., *N. Engl. J. Med.*(1982), **307**, 1225-1230.
91. Baumgartner, J. D., Glauser, M. P., McCutchan, J. A., Ziegler, E. J., Melle, G. V., Klauber, M. R., Vogt, M., Muehlen, E., Luethy, R., Chiolero R., and Geroulanos, S., *Lancet* (1985), **ii**, 59-63.
92. McCutchan, J. A., Wolf, J. L., Ziegler, E. J. and Braude, I. A., *Schweiz. Med. Wschr.* (1983), **113 (Suppl. 14)**, 40-45.
93. Calandra, T., Glauser, M. P., Schellekens, J., Verhoef, J. and The Swiss-Dutch J5 Immunoglobulin Study Group, *J. Infect. Dis.* (1988), **158**, 312-319.
94. Band, J. D., Chamberland, M. E., Platt, T., Weaver, R. E., Thornsberry, C. and Froser, D. W., *J. Infect. Dis.* (1983), **148**, 754-758.

95. Gotschlich, E. C., *In:* Bacterial Vaccines, Germanier, R. (ed.), Academic Press, Orlando, FL, (1984), 237-255.
96. Lapeyssonie, L., *Bull. WHO* (1963), **28 (Suppl.)**, 1-114.
97. Gotschlich, E. C., Goldschneider, I. and Artenstein, M. S., *J. Exp. Med.* (1969), **129**, 1367-1384.
98. Artenstein, M. S., Gold, R., Zimmerly, J. G., Wyle, F. A., Schneider, H. and Harkins, C., *N. Engl. J. Med.* (1970), **282**, 417-420.
99. Mäkelä, P. H., Käyhty, H., Weckström, P., Sivonen, A. and Renkonen, O.-V., *Lancet* (1975), **ii**, 883-886.
100. Wahdan, M. H., Sallam, S. A., Hassan, M. N., Gawad, A. A., Rakha, A. S., Sippel, J. E., Hablas, J. E., Sanborn, W. R., Kassem, N. M., Riad, S. M. and Cvjetanovic, B., *Bull. WHO* (1977), **55**, 645-651.
101. Peltola, H., Mäkelä, P. H., Käyhty, H. M., Jousimies, H., Herva, E., Hällström, K., Sivonen, A., Renkonen, O.-V., Pettay, O., Karanko, V., Ahvonen, P. and Sarna, S., *N. Engl. J. Med.* (1977), **297**, 686-691.
102. Hennings, H. J. and Lugowsky, C., *J. Immunol.* (1981), **127**, 1011-1018.
103. Frasch, C. E., *Vaccine* (1987), **5**, 3-4.
104. Zollinger, W. D., Mandrell, R. E. and Griffis, J. M., *In:* Seminars in Infectious Disease, **Vol. IV**, Robbins, J. B., Hill, J. C. and Sadoff, J. C. (eds.), Thieme-Stratton, New York (1982), 254-262.
105. Frasch, C. E., Coetzee, G., Zahradrik, D. M. and Wang, L. Y., *In:* Pathogenic Neisseria, Schoolnik, G. K. (ed.), American Society for Microbiology, Washington, D.C., (1985), 633-640.
106. Collins, F. M., *In:* Bacterial Vaccines, Germanier, R. (ed.), Academic Press, Orlando, FL, (1984), 373-418.
107. Ferguson, R. G. and Simes, A. B., *Tubercle* (1949), **30**, 5-11.
108. Boyden, S. V., *Br. J. Exp. Pathol.* (1957), **38**, 611-617.
109. Lotte, A., Wasz-Höckert, O., Lert, F., Dumitrescu, N. and Poisson, N., *Dev. Biol. Stand* (1979), **43**, 111-119.
110. Torriani, R., Zimmermann, A. and Morell, A., *Schweiz. Med. Wochenschr.* (1979), **109**, 708-713.
111. Hennessen, W., Freudenstein, H. and Engelhardt, H., *J. Biol. Stand.* (1977), **5**, 139-146.
112. Travers, D.B., *Lancet* (1981), ***i***, 1001-1002.
113. Lu, M. C., Lien, M. H., Becker, R. E., Heine, H. C., Biggs, A. M., Lipovsek, D., Gupta, R., Robbins, P. W., Grosskinsky, C. M., Hubbard, S. C. and Young, R. A., *Infect. Immun.* (1987), **55**, 2378-2382.
114. Moss, B. and Flexner, C., *Ann. Rev. Immunol.* (1987), **5**, 305-324.
115. Leffler, H. and Svanborg-Eden, C., *FEMS Microbiol. Lett.* (1980), **8**, 127-134.
116. Rauss, K., Kétyi, I., Matusovits, E., Szendrei, L., Vertényi, A. and Várbiró, B., *Acta. Microbiol. Acad. Sci. Hung.* (1972), **19**, 19-28.
117. Levine, M. M., Nalin, D. R., Hoover, D. L., Bergquist, E. J., Hornick, R. B. and Young, C. R., *Infect. Immun.* (1979), **23**, 729-736.
118. Levine, M. M., Black, R. E., Brinton, C. C., Jr., Clements, M. L., Fusco, P., Hughes, T. P., O'Donnell, S., Robins-Browne, R., Wood, S. and Young, C. R., *Scand. J. Infect. Dis.* (**Suppl.**), (1982), **33**, 83-95.
119. Evans, D. G., Evans, D. J., Jr., Opekun, A. R. and Graham, D. Y., *In:* Bacterial Vaccines and Local Immunity, Tagliabue, A. ,Rappuoli, R. and Piazzi, S. E. (eds.), Edita Da Sclavo Sp. A., Siena, Italy, (1986), 155-156.
120. Levine, M. M., *In:* Bacterial Vaccines, Germanier, R. (ed.), Academic Press, Orlando, FL, (1984), 187-235.
121. Klipstein, F. A., Engert, R. F. and Houghton, R. A., *Infect. Immun.* (1983), **40**, 888-893.
122. Holmgren, J., *Nature* (1981), **292**, 413-417.
123. Finkelstein, R. A., Sciortino, C. V., Rieke, L. C., Burks, M. F. and Boesman-Finkelstein, M., *Infect. Immun.* (1984), **45**, 518-521.
124. Schmidt, M. A., O'Hanley, P. and Schoolnik, G. K., *In:* Bacterial Vaccines and Local Immunity, Tagliabue, A. , Rappuoli, R. and Piazzi S. E. (eds.), Edita Da Sclavo Sp. A., Siena, Italy. (1986), 389-398.

125. Gotschlich, E. C., *In:* Bacterial Vaccines, Germanier, R. (ed.), Academic Press, Orlando, FL, (1984), 353-371.

126. Kellogg, D. S., Cohen, I. R., Norins, L. C., Schroeter, A. L. and Reising, G., *J. Bacteriol.* (1968), **96**, 596-605.

127. Swanson, J., Kraus, S. J. and Gotschlich, E. C., *J. Exp. Med.* (1971), **134**, 886-906.

128. Greenberg, L., Diena, B. B., Ashton, F. A., Wallace, R., Kenny, C. P., Znamirowski, R., Ferrari, H. and Atkinson, J., *Can. J. Public Health* (1974), **65**, 29-33.

129. Tramont, E. C. and Boslego, J. W., *Vaccine* (1985), **3**, 3-10.

130. Brinton, C. C., Wood, S. W., Brown, A., Labik, A. M., Bryan, A. R., Lu, S. W., Polen, S., Tramont, E. and Sadoff, J., *In:* Seminars in Infectious Disease, **Vol. IV.** Bacterial Vaccines, Robbins, J. B., Hill, J. and Sadoff, J. C. (eds.), Thieme-Stratton, Inc., New York, (1982), 140-159.

131. Schoolnik, G. K., Tai, J. Y. and Gotschlich, E. C., *Prog. Allergy,* (1983), **33**, 314-331.

132. Rothbard, J. B., Fernandez, R., Wand, L., Teng, N. N. H., et al., *Proc. Nat. Acad. Sci. USA* (1985), **2**, 915-919.

133. Blake, M. S., *In:* The Pathogenesis of Bacterial Infections, Jackson, G. G. and Thomas, H. (eds.), Springer-Verlag, Berlin, (1985), 51-66.

134. Buchanan, T. M., Siegel, M. S., Chen, K. C. S. and Pearce, W. A., *In:* Seminars in Infectious Disease, **Vol. IV**. Bacterial Vaccines. Robbins, J. B., Hill, J. and Sadoff, J. C. (eds.), Thieme-Stratton, Inc., New York. (1982), 160-164.

135. Robbins, J. B., Schneerson, R. and Pittman, M., *In:* Bacterial Vaccines, Germanier, R. (ed.), Academic Press, Orlando, FL, (1984), 289-316.

136. Sutton, A., Schneerson, R., Kendall-Morris, S. and Robbins, J. B., *Infect. Immun.* (1982), **35**, 95-104.

137. Peltola, H., Käyhty, H., Sivonen, A. and Mäkelä, P. H., *Pediatrics* (1977), **60**, 730-737.

138. Hendly, J. O., Wenzel, J. G., Ashe, K. M. and Samuelson, J. S., *Pediatrics* (1987), **80**, 351-354.

139. Daum, R. S., Mancuse, E. K. and Giebink, G. S., *Pediatrics* (1988), **81**, 893-897.

140. Granoff, D. M., Schackelford, P. G. and Suarez, B. K., *New Engl. J. Med.* (1986), **315**, 1584-1590.

141. Barkin, R. M., Hendley, J. O., and Zahradnik, J., *Pedriatr. Infect. Dis.* (1987), **6**, 20-23.

142. Käyhty, H., Eskola, J., Peltola, H., Stout, M. G., Samuelson, J. S. and Gordon, L. K., *J. Infect. Dis.* (1987), **155**, 100-106.

143. Anderson, P., Pichichero, M. and Edwards, K., *J. Pediatr.* (1987), **111**, 644-650.

144. Schneerson, R., Barrera, O., Sutton, A. and Robbins, J. B., *J. Exp. Med.* (1980), **152**, 361-370.

145. Lenoir, A. A., Granoff, P. D. and Granoff, D. M., *Pediatrics* (1987), **80**, 283-287.

146. Eskola, J., Peltola, H., Takala, A. K., Käyhty, H., Hakulinen, M., Karanko, V., Kela, E., Rekola, P., Rönnberg, P.-R., Samuelson, J. S., Gordon, L. K. and Mäkelä, P. H., *N. Engl. J. Med.* (1987), **317**, 717-722.

147. Ward, J. I., Brenneman, G., Letson, G. and Heyward, W., Alaska Vaccine Efficacy Trial Study Group, *Abstr. Intersci. Conf. Antimicrob. Agents Chemother.* (1988), **28th, 1988** , 309.

3. Viral Vaccines

Marta Granström

3.1 Measles Vaccine

Etiological Agent and Pathogenesis. Measles, (rubeola) is caused by a *paramyxovirus* first isolated by Enders and Peebles in 1954. This highly contagious disease is transmitted in an aerosol of virus-infected droplets from the respiratory tract. During the prevaccination era, children in industrialized countries generally had a self-limiting disease characterized by conjunctivitis, bronchitis, fever and a rash; complications included pneumonia (mostly bacterial) and encephalitis. A late complication of measles in early childhood is the development of a progressive, fatal neurological disease, termed subacute sclerosing panencephalitis. Death due to complications following measles infection remains one of the leading causes of child mortality in developing countries.

History of Immunization. Two approaches to vaccine development were adopted, one was based on killed (inactivated) strains and the other on live, attenuated strains [1]. The formaldehyde-inactivated, alum-precipitated vaccine was licensed in the United States in 1963 and withdrawn in 1967 because its protective effect was insufficient. In addition, the vaccinees exposed to the wild virus developed atypical measles with fever and rash but also pneumonitis.

The attenuated live vaccine with the Edmonston B strain was also licensed in 1963 in the United States. A large scale field trial in the United Kingdom showed high seroconversion rates, a long antibody response, and a 84-94 % decrease in attack rate among the 36 000 immunized children. Further attenuation of the vaccine strain in chick embryo cells yielded the Schwartz and the Moraten strains. Both strains are included in current measles (and combined measles-mumps-rubella) vaccines. Attenuation of the original Edmonston strain in human diploid cells yielded the Edmonston-Zagreb strain, also in current use [2]. With the introduction of general immunization against measles, the disease has almost disappeared in many countries (see below).

Production and Properties of Measles Vaccines. The attenuated measles vaccine strain is usually grown in primary culture using chick embryo cells or human diploid cells. The WHO requirements for the seed virus and cell substrates are described in [3, p. 52; 4, p. 179]. Tests for monitoring measles vaccine grown in chick embryo cells include tests for nonadsorbing viruses and avian leukosis viruses. For vaccines grown in human diploid cells, chromosomal monitoring requirements have been formulated. Potency is checked by titration of the virus in tissue culture (minimum requirement 1 000 $TCID_{50}$ per human dose). To test for stability, a sample of the final freeze-dried vaccine is incubated at 37 °C for seven days: the sample must then contain at least 1 000 $TCID_{50}$ in each human dose. The vaccine is lyophilized; reconstituted vaccine should be used immediately or stored at 0-10 °C for not more than 8 h.

Immunization Recommendations. The vaccine is given at the age of 15-24 months [5] or even younger in developing countries [2]. In the US and many European countries, a combined measles-mumps-rubella (MMR) is usually given (see section 3.4). As for all live vaccines, immunization of immunocompromised individuals is not generally recommended. Immunization of pregnant women should be avoided although no increased risks have been documented for measles vaccine.

Adverse Reactions. Current attenuated measles strains give a few mild reactions, mostly consisting of fever and rash 7-10 days after immunization. The neurologic reaction of the Guillian-Barré syndrome has been reported but is extremely rare.

Vaccine Efficacy. The rapid decrease of measles morbidity in the US after introduction of general immunization is a good example of vaccine efficacy [5, 6]. Over a period of 20 years the rate of notified cases fell by more than 99 %. Subacute sclerosing panencephalitis also decreased. The overall protective efficacy of the current strains is 90 % but is lower in children of 12 months of age due to the presence of maternal antibody. Life-long immunity after one dose of vaccine has not been proven. Increased disease incidence in the US has raised the question of the possible need for a two-dose schedule [5]. A second dose administered at age 4-6 years [5a] or at age 11-12 years [5b] as combined vaccine has recently been recommended by US health authorities.

Future Prospects. Given the efficacy and acceptability of the currently used attenuated measles strains, there has been little incentive for vaccine development. However current vaccines are not very stable at high temperature, which is a concern in many developing countries. Furthermore, a large proportion of morbidity and mortality in children in developing countries occurs before the recommended age for immunization. Research is centered on solving these two problems. More immunogenic strains and/or higher doses of attenuated vaccines are being investigated [2]. Another approach would be to renew work on the development of a killed (inactivated) vaccine. Inactivated vaccines have so far failed. This is probably the result of a lack of neutralizing antibodies to the viral fusion surface protein that is destroyed in the inactivation process [7]. Subunit vaccines based on the hemagglutinin and the fusion proteins of measles virus have successfully been tested in animals and may provide a vaccine especially suited for developing countries [8].

3.2 Mumps Vaccine

Etiological Agent and Pathogenesis. Mumps is caused by a member of the *paramyxovirus* group and is also known as (epidemic) parotitis due to its predominant symptom of infection of the salivary (parotid) gland. Transmission occurs via infected aerosol droplets. The disease is generally characterized by moderate fever and swelling of the salivary glands. Subclinical infection occurs in ca. one third of infected individuals. Most cases occur in children 5-10 years of age. The most frequent complication is meningoencephalitis, giving clinical symptoms in >10 % of patients. Orchitis, a less common but feared complication in postpubertal males, results in impairment of fertility in 10-20 % of cases but absolute sterility is rare.

History of Immunization. Isolation of the causative agent for mumps by Habel, 1945 from chick embryo was followed by attenuation studies for vaccine development. Development of an inactivated (killed) vaccine, was also initiated; a killed vaccine was licensed in the US in 1950-1978 but has low long-term protective efficacy [9]. An inactivated mumps vaccine was also produced in Finland for immunizing military recruits; it decreased disease incidence by 94 % [10]. Immunization with an attenuated mumps vaccine (Jeryl Lynn strain cultured in chick embryo cells) licensed in 1967 in the United States resulted in a 97 % decline of disease incidence in the general population by 1981 [i, 11, 12]. Chick embryonic cells are used to propagate another highly attenuated strain, Urabe Am9, developed in Japan [13]. The Rubini strain, developed in Switzerland, is used in a vaccine in which the virus is grown in human diploid cells [14]. Vaccines based on the Leningrad-3 strain have been used in the Soviet Union and other countries since 1974.

Production and Characterization of Mumps Vaccines. The WHO requirements for the above-mentioned live mumps vaccine have recently been formulated [15, p. 139]. Controls, thermostability tests, and requirements are as for measles vaccines, i.e., the minimum potency should be retained after inoculation for one week at 37 °C (see section 3.1). No minimum requirement of potency has been established by the WHO but a commonly used minimum dosage is 5 000 $TCID_{50}$ per human dose. The vaccine is lyophilized, reconstituted vaccine should be used without delay.

Immunization Recommendations. Mumps vaccine is recommended to be given to all susceptible individuals over the age of 12 months [16]. It is usually given in combination with measles and rubella vaccines in industrialized countries (see section 3.4). A two-dose schedule with combined vaccine has recently been recommended in the US (see measles vaccine).

Vaccine Efficacy. Clinical efficacy is 75-90 % for the live vaccine containing the Jeryl Lynn strain [12]. Similar results have been shown for the other strains or inferred from serologic comparisons. The long-term protective efficacy of the inactivated mumps vaccine used in Finland has not been established but antibody responses indicate that it may give a shorter-term immunity than a live vaccine due to a lack of antibody response to the fusion protein [17] as in the case of the inactivated measles vaccine (see section 3.7).

Adverse Reactions. Mumps vaccine is one of the least reactogenic attenuated vaccines. Side effects are rare and mild. No cases of atypical mumps were found after immunization of Finnish recruits with killed mumps vaccine [17]. Mumps meningitis following immunization with an alternated, combined vaccine containing the Urabe strain has recently been reported [xx].

Future Prospects. The present vaccine is highly satisfactory and little effort has been devoted to further development. Subunit vaccines based on the hemagglutinin neuraminidase and the fusion surface proteins of mumps virus are protective in animal models [18].

3.3 Rubella Vaccine

Etiological Agent and Pathogenesis. Rubella also known as German measles, is caused by a member of the *togavirus* group. The virus was isolated in 1962 by two independent American groups. In 1941 Gregg reported that this mild disease could cause severe congenital cataract in children born to mothers who were infected during the first trimester of pregnancy. Transmission of the virus occurs by the respiratory route. The clinical picture is a discrete rash and low grade fever. 25-50 % of cases remain subclinical. Arthritis is a common complication; encephalitis is less common than in measles or varicellae (1/6 000 cases). The congenital rubella syndrome is usually characterized by hearing impairment, ocular lesions, cardiac malformation, microcephaly, and mental retardation. The severity of defects is related to fetal age at the time of maternal infection, with the most severe damage seen after infection during the first month of pregnancy.

History of Immunization. Live attenuated rubella vaccines were licensed in several countries in 1969-1970. One of the first vaccines contained the Cendehill strain, grown in rabbit kidney cells [19]. Other vaccines were based on the HPV-77 strain grown in either duck embryo cultures or in dog kidney cultures. The latter vaccine produced arthritis symptoms in 50-60 % of adult female vaccinees as compared to 10-20 % for the other two vaccines. A vaccine based on the RA 27/3 strain, isolated and propagated in human diploid cells, was licensed in the mid-1970s in Europe and in 1979 in the US [20]. This vaccine gave a better immune response and had less side effects than the other vaccines. It has replaced other rubella strains in the current vaccines.

Production and Properties of Rubella Vaccines. The attenuated RA 27/3 strain is grown in human diploid cells. The WHO requirements for rubella vaccine include control of normal karology of the human diploid cells [21, p. 54; 22, p. 313]. The minimal potency requirement, determined by titration in tissue culture, is 1 000 $TCID_{50}$ per human dose. The vaccine is lyophilized; reconstituted vaccine should be used immediately or stored at 2-8 °C for not more than 8 h.

Immunization Recommendations. Vaccination strategies range from protection of the individual as in the U.K. (until recently) to indirect protection as in the US [23, 24]. Protection is achieved by general immunization of adolescent girls, usually combined with post partum vaccination of seronegative women. Indirect protection of adult women by immunization of young children is often combined with vaccination of seronegative women.

A combination of these strategies is used in some European countries, e.g. Sweden [25]. This program includes routine screening of all pregnant women, post partum vaccination of seronegatives, and two-dose immunization of children with combined measles-mumps-rubella vaccine. Although the risks for the fetus seem small, the vaccine should not be given to pregnant women and contraceptive measures are recommended for three months after immunization. A two-dose schedule with combined vaccine has recently been recommended in the US (see measles vaccine).

Adverse Reactions. The currently used RA 27/3 strain has few and mild side effects. The joint manifestations, mainly arthralgia, are more common in adults. Intrauterine infections during pregnancy have been documented for all three strains (Ce HPV-77 and RA 27/3 [26]. No abnormalities related to congenital rubella inf have been documented for any of the strains.

Vaccine Efficacy. The efficacy of the current strain is ca. 90 %. The incide congenital rubella virus infection decreased in countries with a routine immunization program against the disease. The duration of immunity, has not yet been determined. The risks to the fetus upon a maternal reinfection are also unknown and may be very small.

Future Prospects. The current vaccine is considered safe and efficient and no efforts are devoted to further development.

3.4 Combined Measles-Mumps-Rubella-Vaccine

History of Immunization. The first combined measles-mumps-rubella (MMR) vaccine was licensed in the US in 1971. It contains the Moraten measles strain (section 3.1) the Jeryl Lynn mumps strain (section 3.2), both grown in chick embryo cultures and the RA 27/3 rubella strain (section 3.3) grown in human diploid cells. Three other combined vaccines were licensed later and are also in current use. The triple vaccine has replaced the monovalent vaccines used in general immunization programs for children in the US and in many European countries.

Production and Properties of Combined Vaccines. The minimum potencies for the attenuated strains of measles, mumps, and rubella virus are the same as in the monovalent vaccines, i.e., >1 000 $TCID_{50}$ for measles, >5 000 $TCID_{50}$ for mumps and >1 000 $TCID_{50}$ for rubella. The vaccine is lyophilized and should be stored at 2-8 °C.

Immunization Recommendations. In many countries, one dose of vaccine is administered to children at the age of 15-24 months. Two doses are given in some European countries [25] and are also recommended in the US since 1989 (see measles vaccine). In Sweden, a first dose is administered at 18 months and a second at 12 years of age, replacing the monovalent programs for measles and rubella immunization respectively. In the US, the combination of MMR with oral polio vaccine and diphtheria-tetanus-pertussis (DTP) at 15 months has been recommended [27, 28].

Adverse Reactions. The side effects are the same as for the monovalent vaccines, the measles component being the most reactogenic. The rate of adverse reactions is <0.5-4 % [29].

Vaccine Efficacy and Future Prospects. The efficacy of the combined preparation is the same as for the monovalent vaccines with an overall efficacy of 90-95 % [6]. The life-long protective efficacy of a single injection has not been proven. Further combinations with an attenuated varicella component are currently under investigation [30].

3.5 Polio Vaccine

Etiological Agent and Pathogenesis. Polio (infantile paralysis) is caused by a *picornavirus* of the genus *enterovirus*. A poliovirus strain was first isolated in cell culture by Enders, Weller and Robbins in 1949. In 1951, polio virus isolates were officially grouped into three serotypes, type 1 (Brunhilde), type 2 (Lansing) and type 3 (Leon). Transmission is mainly via the oral - fecal route and the virus reaches the central nervous system by way of the blood stream. The vast majority of infections are subclinical. The non-paralytic disease has a mild or minor form with fever and general malaise and a more severe or major form with additional symptoms of meningitis/meningoencephalitis. Paralytic polio, with its most severe bulbar form, is estimated to represent 5-10 % of clinical cases. The mortality rate is 5-10 % of clinical cases, i.e., 1-2 % of all infections. Severe paralysis is seen in 10-20 % of clinical cases, mild or moderate paralysis in 30 %.

With improved sanitation and standards of living, a shift towards infection at a higher age was observed in industrialized countries in the prevaccination era. During the first half of this century, peak incidence was noted in the age group 5-14 years. A large proportion of cases occurred in young adults. In the developing countries, polio has maintained its character of infantile paralysis with the majority of children being infected during the first few years of life. Cases of paralytic polio occur only in the youngest age groups.

History of Immunization. The first large scale field trial of an inactivated (killed) polio vaccine was launched in the US in the early 1950s only a few years after successful propagation of the virus in tissue culture. Inactivated polio vaccine (IPV) was licensed for general use in the US in 1955 [31, 32]. In 1955 cases of atypical paralytic polio were reported, most of them were associated with two lots of vaccine from Cutter [33]. Although live poliovirus was recovered from vaccine supplied by other manufacturers, this failure of inactivation is known as the Cutter incident. The total toll was 269 cases, of which 192 were paralytic (with ten deaths). Clinical trials with a live attenuated oral polio vaccine (OPV) were started in 1958 and the vaccine was licensed in the US in 1962 [34, 35]. Immunization with OPV alone has been used from the late 1950s - early 1960s in Europe. One of the largest immunization campaigns was launched in the Sovjet Union in 1960 when OPV was given to ca. 77×10^6 people. A few European countries have used only IPV [36, 38]. In Sweden, clinical trials with IPV were started in 1953 and general immunization was introduced in 1957 [36]. All three strategies were effective in reducing the incidence of paralytic polio. With IPV alone, an 80 % reduction rate was achieved in the US with less than 50 % of the population immunized [31, 32, 34]. The decrease of polio continued at the same rate after introduction of OPV. Introduction of the massive IPV campaign in Sweden resulted in a 93 % decrease of paralytic disease after six years of immunization [36].

Production and Properties of Polio Vaccines. Oral polio vaccines are manufactured with the attenuated Sabin strains. Inactivated polio vaccines are mostly produced with the type 1 Mahoney strain, type 2 MEF-1 strain and type 3 Saukett strain. Primary and secondary monkey (*Cynomolgus*) kidney cultures or human diploid cells are most commonly used for culture. The WHO requirements for both OPV and IPV produced in primary monkey kidney cells include tests

1) for the absence of cytopathogenic viruses with the exception of some foamy viruses [4, p. 40; 39, p. 107; 45, p. 108),

2) the absence of simian B virus in rabbits and

3) the absence of SV_{40} in sensitive cells (usually primary green monkey *Cercopitecus* kidney cultures).

Minimal potency requirements for OPV were formulated by the WHO in 1987 [15, p. 165]. A single human dose of trivalent oral vaccine should contain approximately $10^{5.5}$ - $10^{6.5}$ infectious units of type 1, $10^{4.5}$ - $10^{5.5}$ of type 2, and $10^{5.0}$ - $10^{6.0}$ of type 3. For IPV, recommendations of 40:8:32 D-antigen units per human dose for types 1, 2, and 3 respectively were issued in 1981 [22]. The potency tests for OPV (and IPV prior to inactivation) are performed by titration in tissue culture. *In vivo* potency tests are also required for IPV but neither the animal species nor the number of injections is specified. Inactivation of polio vaccine by formaldehyde is controlled by titration of polio-sensitive cells (usually *Cynomolgus* or *Cercopithecus*) in tissue culture. Oral polio vaccines are supplemented with a stabilizer, usually magnesium chloride or sorbitol. Both OPV and IPV contain antibiotics, usually neomycin; OPV is best stored at -20 °C but can be stored at 2-4 °C for a variable length of time; IPV is stored at 2-8 °C.

Immunization Recommendations. Recommendations vary but at least three doses of OPV are given. In the US, five doses are recommended, in Sweden four and in Finland six. The WHO recommends four doses for infants in developing countries.

Adverse Reactions. Serious adverse reactions of paralytic polio have only been reported for OPV with a predominance for type 3 [32, 40] (incidence = $1/1 \times 10^6$ vaccine recipients including both non-immune and immune individuals). No cases of IPV-induced paralytic polio have been reported after 30 years of use (with the exception of the Cutter incident). IPV is considered to be the least reactogenic of all the vaccines used for childhood immunization.

Vaccine Efficacy. Both OPV and IPV have proven highly efficient in eliminating polio from industrialized countries with general immunization programs. The protective efficacy is close to 100 % after at least three doses of vaccine with adequate immunogenicity. Serologic data reported for OPV from developing countries have been less than encouraging. Both vaccines have eliminated the circulation of wild type strains in industrialized countries with high immunization rates. Outbreaks among groups refusing immunization have occured [31]. In 1984, nine cases of paralytic polio caused by type 3 occurred in Finland [40]. The low immunogenicity of the IPV used in Finland has been known since the late 1960s [41]. The new IPV developed in the Netherlands with its high antigen content is given in European countries in at least three doses [42]. Two doses or even one dose of the new IPV preparations have been claimed to be highly protective. A two dose-schedule has been used in Africa and protective efficiency was ca. 89 % [43]. Inactivated polio vaccine is more heat-stable and can be combined with diphtheria-tetanus-pertussis vaccines.

Future Prospects. Further development of OPV is aimed at reducing production costs by use of microcarrier cell cultures on beads etc. in fermentors [42]. Use of continuous cell lines is being investigated. An IPV produced in a continuous cell line is currently licensed in France [44]. The WHO requirements for production of vaccines in continuous cell lines are formulated [45, p. 93].

3.6 Hepatitis B Vaccine

Etiological Agent and Pathogenesis. Hepatitis B is caused by the hepatitis B virus (HBV), a member of the *hepadna virus* group. The presence of a new antigen called the Australia (Au) antigen, or hepatitis B surface antigen (HBsAg) in the blood of patients with leukemia, Down's syndrome and hepatitis was shown by Blumberg in 1964-1967. Other antigens HBeAg and HBcAg, were described later and correlated with infectivity; they are found in the 42 nm Dane particle, i.e. the infectious virion.

The HBV is a pathogen only for humans but certain monkeys, in particular chimpanzees, are also susceptible to infection. Transmission in humans occurs mainly by inoculation with infected blood. The virus is excreted in body fluids, causing infection through saliva and sexual contacts. A chronic active carrier state is established in 5-10 % of adult cases; chronic hepatitis develops in 25-30 % of the carriers, often leading to cirrhosis of the liver: 90 % of infants infected at birth become carriers. Hepatitis B occurs throughout the world; the incidence varies from < 0.5 % in Western Europe and the US to 5-15 % in Southeast Asia and Southern Africa [46, 47].

Hepatitis B virus plays an important role in hepatocellular carcinoma although the exact mechanism has not yet been determined [46].

History of Immunization. Heat-inactivated HBsAg positive serum was used by Krugman in 1971 to immunize children. A 70 % protection rate was found upon challenge with active virus. The high protective efficacy of hepatitis B vaccine derived from purified, inactivated HBsAg from positive plasma was demonstrated in 1980 [48]. The vaccine, developed in the US, was licensed for general use in 1981. Studies in 1980-1983 also showed that the HBV vaccine in combination with human anti HBV immune globulin (HBIG) prevented development of the carrier state in infants born to carrier mothers. Hepatitis B vaccine, was the first vaccine to be routinely produced by DNA recombinant technology in yeast. Serologic studies indicate that the protective efficacy of the recombinant vaccines is the same as that of the plasma-derived vaccine. Genetically engineered vaccines were licensed in the US in 1986 and subsequently in several European countries.

Production and Properties of Hepatitis B Vaccines. The WHO requirements for plasma-derived HBV specify guidelines for selection of donors of HBsAg-positive plasma [49, p. 70]. The plasma pool must be subjected to extensive tests in animals, fertile eggs and cell cultures for extraneous viruses and *Mycobacterium tuberculosis*. The purified HBsAg (>95 % pure) is inactivated by treatment with pepsin followed by urea (8 mol/l), and formaldehyde or by heat with or without formaldehyde. After controls for purity and antigen content, an alum adjuvant is added; the vaccine must be stored at 5 ± 3 °C. No minimal requirement of antigen content has been formulated but a commonly used vaccine contains 20 μg HBsAg per human dose.

The WHO requirements for HBV made by recombinant DNA technology state that such vaccines may contain the S gene products or the S/pre-S combination [15, p. 106]; licensed recombinant vaccines contain only the S gene product. A full description of the host cell (currently *Saccharomyces cerevisiae*) and the expression vector is required. The HBsAg is commonly purified by precipitation, ultrafiltration and chromatography.

Tests for HBsAg and residual cell or plasmid DNA are required before addition of adjuvant. No animal antigen requirements have been formulated but a potency assay in mice has been outlined. Commonly used recombinant yeast vaccines contain 10 or 20 μg HBsAg per human dose.

Immunization Recommendations. Most Western European countries and the US have issued recommendations for vaccination of risk groups [50-52]. In general, pre-exposure prophylaxis is recommended to medical and other staff in frequent contact with high risk groups or with blood from such groups. Immunization of patient groups frequently receiving blood or blood products, as well as patients in certain institutions is also recommended.

For pre-exposure prophylaxis, three 20 μg doses of plasma-derived vaccine are given at day 0, 30 and 6 months intramuscularly in the deltoid region. Children <11 years of age should receive 5 μg at each injection. Postexposure prophylaxis for infants to HBsAg, HBeAg positive mothers is 0.5 ml intramuscular injection of human antiHBV immune globulin (HBIG) (see section 5.4 Vaccine (10 μg) should be given at birth and then at one and six months of age. For postexposure prophylaxis of adults, 1 ml HBIG should be given immediately together with three doses of vaccine administered as for preexposure prophylaxis.

Adverse Reactions. Side effects are mild and mainly local in <20 % of the vaccinees at the site of injection.

Vaccine Efficacy. The overall vaccine efficacy is 90 % (with no response upon immunization) in 5-10 % of the vaccinees. In individuals with seroconversion to HBsAg, protective efficacy is almost 100 %. Studies on the duration of protection beyond 5-10 years are not yet available. The protective efficacy of HBIG and vaccine administered to newborns born to carrier mothers has been estimated to be more than 90 % [46].

Future Prospects. Current HBV vaccines are safe and have a high efficacy but also high production costs. Research is aimed at the development of cheaper, more immunogenic vaccines. The inclusion of the pre S (P 31) region of the viral genome in addition to the present S (P 25) region is being investigated in yeast-derived recombinant vaccines [53, 54]. Other antigens such as HBcAg are also being studied. Polypeptide vaccines based on the major determinants of HBsAg are undergoing clinical trials. Synthetic peptides may provide the ultimate solution to the problem of immunogenic, readily available HBV vaccines.

3.7 Rabies Vaccine

Etiological Agent and Pathogenesis. Rabies is a lethal disease caused by a neutropic *rhabdovirus* affecting humans and warm-blooded animals. The most common route of transmission to humans is by infected saliva through the bite from a rabid animal. The virus ascends along peripheral nerves to the central nervous system. The incubation period varies from ten days to several months. Symptoms include a nonspecific prodromal stage followed by an acute neurological phase ending in coma and death. The disease is endemic in animals in most parts of the world with some exceptions such as the United Kingdom and parts of Scandinavia [55]. In the urban form, stray dogs and cats act as vectors whereas the sylvatic form involves wild animals. Urban rabies is well-controlled in most countries, but progressive spread of the sylvatic form by foxes is a major problem in Europe. In the US, other animal species are involved, including bats. In Europe and Africa, bats are the vector for an antigenic variant of the virus [56].

History of Immunization. In 1885 Pasteur administered the first vaccination to a young boy who had been bitten by a rabid dog [57]. Serial injections containing a virus strain that had been propagated and attenuated in the spinal cord of rabbits ("fixed" virus) was given in an increasingly virulent form. The treatment was rapidly adopted as standard post exposure prophylaxis. The attenuated vaccine was later replaced by an inactivated (killed) vaccine also produced in neural tissue [57]. However, in some patients the myelin content of the vaccine caused sensitization resulting in neurological disease. An inactivated vaccine produced in duck embryos decreased the risk of neural tissue sensitization. The most widely used rabies vaccine in Europe and in the US was developed in the 1960s and is produced in human diploid cells. A highly purified concentrated duck embryo vaccine is also available. Other vaccines are produced in primary animal cells and continuous cell lines, non-human primate diploid cells are used in the US.

Production and Properties of Rabies Vaccines. Attenuated strains of rabies virus are grown in tissue culture or embryonated duck eggs (see above). The virus suspension is usually concentrated and in some cases purified. Only inactivated vaccines are allowed for human use. Inactivation is mostly achieved by treatment with β-propiolactone, but phenol, formaldehyde or ultraviolet irradiation are also used. The WHO has established requirements for controls of the cells used for virus propagation [15, p. 167; 22, p. 54]. The potency of the vaccine is determined in a mouse challenge assay (minimal requirement 2.5 IU per human dose). The vaccine is then usually lyophilized although adjuvanted preparations are also in use.

Immunization Recommendations. The recommendations vary by vaccine and country. As pre-exposure prophylaxis, three 1 ml doses are usually recommended on days 0, 7 and 28 or on days 0, 28 and 90 (or 365) as 1 ml intramuscular injections in the deltoid or supracapular region [55, 58]. As post-exposure prophylaxis, recommended measures include local wound care, administration of vaccine, and administration of human rabies immune globulin (HRIG, 20 IU per kg of body weight; see also section 5.3). Purified equine rabies immune globulin (40 IU per kg) is used in many developing countries with few side effects [59]. Post exposure vaccine prophylaxis is given in five

1 ml doses on days 0, 3, 7, 14, and 28 by intramuscular injection in previously unimmunized individuals. In individuals who have received pre-exposure prophylaxis, two doses are given on days 0 and 3. Children under four years of age receive 0.5 ml injections.

Vaccine Efficacy. The protective efficacy of the human diploid cell vaccine given (with HRIG) as post exposure prophylaxis was first documented in field trials conducted in Iran in 1974-1975; the survival rate was 100 %. Other studies have confirmed the protective effect of pre- and postexposure immunization with this vaccine. The general opinion that post-exposure vaccine prophylaxis in combination with immune globulin convey 100 % protection has been challenged by two cases of vaccine failure [60]. In other vaccines, a high protective efficacy has been proven in field trials or inferred from comparative serologic studies.

Adverse Reactions. The most common side effects are local redness and induration at the injection site and fever. Desquieting episodes of a serum sickness-like reaction upon repeated immunization have been reported [61] and are possibly due to a sensitizing complex-formation between β-propiolactone and human serum albumin [62] or to the high content of bovine serum residues in the vaccine [63].

Future Prospects. Work is centered on the development of large-scale vaccine production techniques to decrease the high costs and thereby increase availability in poorer countries. One such approach is the use of microcarrier culture systems in fermentors [42]. A vaccine produced in this manner in a continuous cell line is currently being evaluated. A subunit vaccine based on the surface glycoprotein of the virus is a further possibility. The peptide segment of the glycoprotein that induces the production of neutralizing antibodies has been identified and synthesized. A synthetic peptide vaccine may therefore be the most attractive future alternative [64].

3.8 Influenza Vaccine

Etiological Agent and Pathogenesis. Influenza is caused by two antigenically distinct members of the *orthomyxovirus* group influenza viruses A and B. In 1934 Andrews managed to transfer the influenza A virus from human material to ferrets and later to mice. In 1940, Francis and Magill independently isolated influenza B virus by transmission to ferrets. The virus was subsequently propagated in embryonated hen's eggs and tissue culture. The disease is transmitted by droplet infection from the respiratory tract; it is characterized by high fever, muscle pain and a dry cough. Pneumonia is the main cause of mortality in elderly people and persons with chronic underlying diseases. Influenza occurs worldwide with regular epidemics during the winter months. The recurrent epidemics are caused by small changes (antigenic drift) in the main pathogenic determinants of the virus, i.e. hemagglutinin and neuraminidase. Large pandemics occurr at 10-20 year intervals and are due to substantial changes (antigenic shift) in the pathogenic determinants. Antigenic drift is seen in both influenza A and B whereas antigenic shift has only been noted in influenza A [65].

History of Immunization. The first influenza vaccines produced in hens' eggs were tested in humans in the early 1940s. These inactivated whole virus vaccines had a low content of viral antigens and a high content of contaminating egg protein. Consequently the protective effect was low and the rate of adverse reactions high. Whole virus vaccines purified by ultracentrifugation showed clearly improved immunogenicity and a decreased rate of side reactions. Zonal centrifugation further improved the vaccine for adults but still caused adverse reactions in children. Disruption of influenza vaccine with detergent was used to develop split vaccines in the mid 1960s. Subunit vaccines introduced in the mid 1980s contain concentrated and purified hemagglutinin and neuraminidase [65]. The development of live, attenuated virus strains was pursued in the Soviet Union by serial passages in hens' eggs [65]. However, doubt was cast on their stability. More stable attenuated vaccines were obtained by isolation of temperatur-sensitive and cold-adopted mutants [66]. These strains were successfully tested in humans in the late 1970s but are not in general use. Attenuated vaccines, based on avian-human recombinant strains, are being evaluated in clinical trials.

Production and Properties of Influenza Vaccines. The most commonly used influenza vaccines are of the whole or split virus type. The strains used are specified in annual WHO recommendations. The virus is grown in embryonated hens' eggs (usually pathogen-free) and the allantoic fluid is harvested. According to the WHO requirements, the inactivation method used (usually addition of formaldehyde or β-propriolactone) should inactivate avian leukosis viruses and *mycoplasma* [67, p. 148]. The virus is concentrated and purified by high-speed centrifugation either before or after inactivation. Effective inactivation is controlled by inoculation of embryonated hens' eggs. Hemagglutinin content is usually checked by single radial immunodiffusion against a WHO standard. Whole virus and split virus vaccines usually contain 10-15 μg hemagglutinin per human dose. The inactivated vaccines are usually supplemented with a preservative and stored at 2-8 °C.

The WHO requirements for attenuated (live) vaccines stipulate that pathogen-free eggs must be used. The absence of other pathogens must be controlled in tissue cultures and animals [67, p. 171]. Vaccine potency is determined by titration in embryonated eggs. No minimal requirements of infective dose have been formulated.

Immunization Recommendations. Most countries have recommendations for yearly immunization of high-risk groups. Several countries and the WHO recommend vaccination of all individuals over 65 years. In the US, immunization of children with chronic pulmonary or cardiac disorders or with other chronic diseases residing in institutional care is recommended; 0.25 and 0.5 ml of split virus vaccine are given in the age groups 6-35 months and 3-12 years respectively [68]. For individuals older than 12 years, 0.5 ml of vaccine is recommended.

Adverse Reactions. The incidence of systemic (febrile) and local reactions is <10 % and <20 % respectively for the whole virus vaccines and split vaccines, respectively. An increased rate of the neurological reaction of Guillian-Barré's syndrome was reported in the US after large scale immunization against swine influenza in 1976.

Protective Efficacy. The protective efficacy of influenza vaccines is controversial. Discrepancies are probably due to different vaccines, number of injections given, the age groups under study and occurrence of antigenic drift during the study period. The newer purified whole virus and split virus vaccines are considered to be 70-90 %

effective in healthy adults. The duration of protection is largely dependent on the degree of the antigenic drift. In the case of antigenic shift, little or no protection can be expected. The immune response and protective efficacy in children receiving chemotherapy and in debilitated elderly persons are lower [69]. The protective efficacy in preventing death has been estimated at 74 % [70].

Future Prospects. Research on influenza vaccines is directed toward the synthesis of the hemagglutinin and the neuraminidase antigens and the improvement of their immunogenicity [64]. Another line of development is the attenuated live vaccine approach [66].

3.9 Varicella Vaccine

Etiological Agent and Pathogenesis. The varicella-zoster virus, a member of the *herpes virus* group, causes two distinct clinical manifestations - varicella and herpes zoster [71]. Varicella, also known as chickenpox, is the primary infection. Herpes zoster is caused by the reactivation of the latent varicella virus in ganglion tissue. Varicella is usually a mild infection characterized by a vesicular rash. Transmission occurs by droplet infection from the respiratory tract and by direct contact with vesicle fluid. Complications are encephalitis (1/100-1/300 cases) and pneumonia. The disease occurs worldwide, with 90-95 % of cases occuring before the age of 15 years. Suspected cases of congenital varicella have been described mainly after varicella during the first trimester of pregnancy. Neonatal varicella with a 30 % mortality rate occurs with maternal varicella within one week prior to term without prophylaxis. Varicella in the compromised host is a severe disease with a 10-20 % mortality rate. Herpes zoster, a localized, often painful, vesicular rash is most common in the elderly; it occurs in 10 % of the population.

History of Immunization. The varicella-zoster virus was first isolated and propagated in tissue culture by Weller and Stoddard in 1952. Attenuated, live varicella vaccine was developed in Japan in 1970 using the Oka strain [72]. After serial passages, the attenuated strain was adapted to human diploid cell cultures. The immunogenicity and protective efficacy of the vaccine in healthy children has been demonstrated [72, 73]. Efficacy of the vaccine in children with malignant disease, in particular leukemia, has also been shown [74]. The Oka strain is currently used for vaccine production in Japan, Europe, and the US.

Production and Properties of Varicella Vaccines. The attenuated, live Oka strain is propagated in human diploid cell cultures. The WHO requirements include control for the absence of adventitious agents and the usual conditions for culture in human diploid cells [49, p. 102]. No minimal potency requirements have yet been formulated. Varying doses have been used in clinical trials. The most common formulation is >2 000 plaque forming units per human dose. The vaccine is lyophilized; reconstituted vaccine should be used without delay.

Immunization Recommendations. Varicella vaccine is not yet recommended for general immunization in Europe or the US. It is given to children with leukemia during remission or when chemotherapy is withheld for one week prior to and after vaccination [74]. A second dose is often given to children who remain seronegative after the first injection.

Adverse Reactions. Local swelling and pain occured in 1-5 % of healthy children and ca. 20 % of adults. Systemic reactions with fever and a rash are reported in 5-10 % of both healthy children and adults. Fever and rash occurred in 40 % of vaccine recipients with chemotherapy suspended for two weeks.

Vaccine Efficacy. Protective efficacy in healthy children is 95-100 % with persistence of immunity over a 5-10 year period. In adults, protective efficacy is 60-80 %, and possibly of shorter duration. In children with malignancies, protective efficacy is 60-92 %. Spread from vaccine-induced vesicular rash has been documented in household contacts.

Future Prospects. The currently investigated, attenuated Oka strain vaccine is effective but long-term immunity and zoster incidence remain to be established. The problem of latency and of vaccine-induced rash could be overcome by the development of a subunit vaccine produced either by a recombinant DNA technique or by using synthetic peptides.

3.10 Yellow Fever Vaccine

Etiological Agent and Pathogenesis. Yellow fever is a hemorrhagic fever caused by a member of the *togavirus* group [75, 76]. The virus was transmitted to rhesus monkeys by Mathis and coworkers in 1927. The virus strain was then propagated by serial passages of intracerebral inoculations in white mice. Yellow fever is transmitted by mosquitoes of the genus *Haemagogus* in South America and of the genus *Aedes* in Africa. The animal reservoir is mainly monkeys. Subclinical infections are common. The incubation period in clinical cases is 3-6 days; symptoms range from transient fever and headache to high fever with meningoencephalitis, followed by jaundice and hemorrhagic manifestations. In the malignant form all these symptoms are present and death occurs within one week. Mortality rates are 40-50 % in the severe forms of the disease.

History of Immunization. Two types of attenuated vaccine were developed in the early 1930s cultured in neural tissue vaccine (Dakar vaccine) and in chick embryo [77]. Initially, both types were given together with human immune serum. In the late 1930s, the vaccine cultured in neural tissue was used for mass immunization in Senegal and the chick embryo vaccine was tested in Brazil. The vaccines were administrered by scarification using normal human serum as stabilizer. The chick embryo cultured vaccine (first the 17E vaccine and later the 17D vaccine) has been most widely used. Numerous problems and accidents were associated with both vaccines. The human serum used as stabilizer caused hepatitis affecting many vaccinees in the armed forces during World War II. Systemic reactions were common. Severe postvaccination encephalitis with a high mortality rate occurred mainly with the neural tissue cultured vaccine. This reaction (mostly in children < one year of age) was also reported with some lots of the 17D vaccine with increased neurotropism; furthermore loss of protective efficacy was noted in tropical climates due to low thermostability. The 17D vaccine in current use is the result of development aimed at careful definition of the properties of the seed virus and at improved thermostability [78].

Production and Properties of Yellow Fever Vaccines. Only certain institutes are approved by the WHO for production of yellow fever vaccine [22, p. 34]. The seed lot virus, usually a substrain of 17D-204, has to be shown to be free from neurotropism by testing in monkeys [45, p. 113; 79, p. 23]. Most producers use seed lots that are free of leukosis virus for production but their use is not mandatory. Virus-infected embryos are harvested, homogenized and the supernatant is used as vaccine. Several tests for adventitious agents are performed. Virus titrations are performed in a mouse assay with a minimal potency requirement of 100 LD_{50} per human dose. The vaccines are lyophilized in the presence of stabilizer. Most current vaccines retain the minimal requirement for two weeks at 22 °C. A vaccine stable for two weeks at 37 °C is requested by WHO for use in tropical areas.

Immunization Recommendations. Vaccination of visitors to endemic areas in equatorial Africa and northern parts of South America is recommended. Immunization is mandatory in several countries for visitors from endemic areas. One 0.5 ml injection is given to both adults and children for both primary and booster immunization. Booster injections are recommended every ten years. The vaccine is not recommended for children under one year of age or for pregnant women.

Adverse Reactions. Yellow fever vaccines are safe and induce only minor local reactions. Transient headache can occur.

Protective Efficacy. Current vaccines are estimated to be 90-95 % protective. Immunization has decreased or eliminated the disease in many endemic areas.

3.11 Tick-Borne Encephalitis Vaccine

Etiological Agent and Pathogenesis. The tick-born encephalitis virus, a member of the *togavirus* group, was first isolated in the Soviet Union in 1937 [76]. Two antigenically distinct forms of the virus cause the disease in Europe and in Eastern USSR. The main vector for the European form is *Ixodes ricinus* and for the Eastern form *I. peruculatus.* Many wild and domestic animals can be infected; the main animal reservoirs are small mammals such as field mice. Transmission is usually by tick bite but infection can occur by drinking untreated cow milk. The incubation period is 7-14 days before onset of fever and malaise. After a 1-2 week recovery period, a second stage with fever and neurological symptoms can follow: meningitis (40 % of cases), meningoencephalitis (40 %) and severe meningoencephalomyelitis (20 %). Mortality rates are 1-2 % in the European form and 20-25 % in the Eastern form, neurological sequelae are seen in 15-40 % of cases. The disease is subclinical or abortive with only the first stage in 75 % of infections. Tick-borne encephalitis is endemic in Central Europe, in the Balkan countries, and in Finland and Sweden.

History of Immunization. The first inactivated (killed) vaccine was developed and used in humans in the USSR in 1939 followed by an attenuated, live vaccine in the

1960s [80]. An inactivated vaccine, developed in Europe with a virus strain isolated from a tick in Austria was subjected to clinical trials in 1973 [81]. The vaccine currently used in Western Europe is a purified, concentrated version of this.

Production and Properties of a Tick-Borne Encephalitis Vaccine. The inactivated vaccine is produced by propagation of the virus in hens' eggs, followed by purification by continuous flow zonal ultracentrifugation and inactivation with formaldehyde. No WHO requirements have been formulated. The vaccine contains not less than 25 protective doses per human dose assayed in a mouse protection test. Human albumin is used as stabilizer and aluminium hydroxide as adjuvant.

Immunization Recommendations. In Austria and Bavaria, immunization of children older than one year is recommended. Other endemic countries recommended immunization of forest workers and other high risk groups. Primary immunization consists of two 0.5 ml intramuscular injections at 1-3 month interval, followed by a third 0.5 ml dose 9-12 months after the second. Booster injections are recommended every three years.

Adverse Reactions. Local and systemic reactions are rare and mild. Low grade fever is occasionally seen, mainly in children after the first injection.

Protective Efficacy. The vaccine is at least 95 % protective against all European virus strains in children and young adults. Seroconversion rates of about 90 % are reported for persons over 65 years of age.

3.12 Japanese Encephalitis Vaccine

Etiological Agent and Pathogenesis. The Japanese encephalitis virus, belonging to the *togavirus* group, was first isolated in 1935 in Japan [75]. The disease is transmitted by the mosquito *Culex tritaeniorhynchus*; the main animal reservoirs are pigs and birds. The incubation period is 5-15 days. The disease is subclinical in at least 95 % of infections. In clinical cases symptoms vary from a mild febrile disease with headache to severe encephalitis. Paralytic forms more commonly affect the upper extremities. In endemic areas the disease affects mainly younger children but also elderly people with mortality rates of 50 %. Neurological sequelae have been reported in 30-40 % of survivors of the severe clinical forms.

History of Immunization. A formaldehyde-killed vaccine, consisting of a 5 % suspension of infected mouse brain tissue, was introduced for human use in Japan in 1954 [82]. The vaccine (Nakayama strain) has been purified by protamine sulfate precipitation since the late 1950s and by absorption with charcoal or kaolin since the early 1960s. A productive efficacy of 80-90 % for the vaccine was shown. The highly purified, mouse brain cultured vaccine produced in Japan is also used for immunizing travellers to endemic areas. In China, a vaccine produced in primary hamster kidney cells has been extensively used since the late 1950s.

Production of Properties of Japanese Encephalitis Vaccines. Several Japanese manufacturers produce the purified vaccine from cultures of mouse neural tissue by similar methods. No WHO requirements have been formulated. A vaccine used for immunizing travellers to endemic areas is prepared by infecting mouse brain with the Nakayama strain. The brain homogenate is purified by protamine sulfate treatment and then inactivated with formaldehyde. Further purification involves ultracentrifugation on a sucrose density gradient. The vaccine is lyophilized; the reconstituted vaccine must be used immediately.

Immunization Recommendations. Primary immunization consists of subcutaneous injection of two 1 ml doses at a 1-2 week interval. A third 1 ml dose is recommended one month later as is a regular booster injection every 1-3 years. Extensive immunization in endemic areas has been considered by the WHO. Children less than three years of age should receive 0.5 ml doses. Immunization is generally recommended for health care workers and other people with extended stay in endemic areas.

Adverse Reactions. Only a few mild, local and systemic reactions have been reported.

Protective Efficacy. Immunization has drastically reduced disease incidence in Japan. The protective efficacy of the current vaccines is estimated to be 90-95 % from serologic studies. A recent placebo-controlled, blinded, randomized trial with two killed vaccines, one containing the Nakayama strain alone and the other in addition the Beijing strain, demonstrated an equal 91 % efficacy for both vacines [83].

3.13 Smallpox Vaccine

Smallpox (variola) was caused by a member of the *pox virus* group, which also includes the vaccinia virus used for immunization. The disease was one of the most devastating infections in human history. Eradication of smallpox is the success story of immunization. In 1967 the WHO launched a massive eradication program - smallpox was still reported from 42 countries. In May 1980, WHO officially declared the world free from smallpox. No proven cases of variola have occurred in the past decade.

Two types of vaccine were manufactured, calf lymph vaccine and egg vaccine [84, p. 6]. Both liquid and lyophilized forms were used. Requirements for manufacturing, control and potency were last formulated by the WHO in 1966. Immunization by multiple puncture with a bifurcated needle was most commonly used. Severe adverse reactions included postvaccination encephalitis and disseminated vaccinia.

General immunization against smallpox was withdrawn in most European countries in the mid 1970s. Requirement for smallpox vaccination was abandoned for international travel in 1982.

Recommendations for civilian immunization in the US include only laboratory workers handling variola virus or other closely related orthopox viruses. Military personnel in the United States and the Soviet Union are routinely vaccinated against smallpox [85].

3.14 Adenovirus Vaccine

Adenoviruses (ADV) are DNA viruses constituting an own group. Over 30 types are recognized, causing a wide panorama of clinical manifestations such as asymptomatic infections, diarrheal disease, epidemic keratoconjunctivitis and upper respiratory infections. Adenovirus types 4, 7 and 21 cause upper respiratory infections with low incidence rates in the general population but with high rates in military recruits [86].

Vaccine development for military personnel led to the successful production of inactivated (killed) vaccine against types 4 and 7 in the mid 1950s. Further research resulted in the development of live, attenuated enteric-coated vaccine to types 4 and 7 with high protective efficacy [86]. A similar vaccine was also developed for type 21 [87]. Military personnel in the United States is routinely immunized with the enteric-coated ADV vaccine to types 4 and 7.

3.15 Rift Valley Fever Vaccine

Rift Valley fever is an arthropod-borne disease known only in Africa [75, 76]. It is caused by a member of the *Bunya virus* group. The major vectors are mosquitoes (*Culex theileri* and *Aedes cabbalus*). The main natural hosts are sheep, cattle, and goats. The incubation period is 2-6 days. Rift Valley fever is a febrile disease with headache and abdominal pain lasting less than one week. Hemorrhagic fever with liver necrosis and encephalitis are the severe manifestations causing mortality and sequelae. Outbreaks occurred in Africa during the 1970s, with the largest outbreak in Egypt in 1977-78.

An inactivated (killed) vaccine (NDBR-103) was produced by the US army in 1967 [88]. The Entebbe strain of the virus was grown in primary monkey kidney cells, inactivated with formaldehyde and lyophilized. The adverse reactions are few and mild. One case of Guillian-Barré occurred in a Swedish military vaccinee [89]. Seroconversion rates after subcutaneous injection of three 1 ml doses given at 1-2 weeks intervals were over 95 %. A new vaccine (GSD-200) based on a cloned version of the original seed virus (Entebbe strain) and grown in diploid rhesus monkey cells is currently undergoing clinical studies. The WHO has formulated requirements for inactivated Rift Valley fever vaccines produced in primary monkey kidney cells and in human or non-human primate diploid cells [4, p. 104]. No minimal potency requirements have been formulated.

3.16 Hepatitis A Vaccine

Epidemic hepatitis or hepatitis A is caused by a small RNA virus belonging to the *picornavirus* group. Hepatitis A virus (HAV) was first identified by electron microscopy in 1973 by Feinstone and coworkers [90]. The propagation of the virus in tissue culture, reported by Provost and Hillerman in 1979 [91], represented a major step towards vaccine development. Transmission of the virus is mainly by the oral-fecal route. After a first replication phase in the gut, the virus replicates in the liver and is excreted by the biliary system into the gut. Maximal fecal HAV excretion occurs some 7 days prior to onset of jaundice and usually ceases at the onset of clinical symptoms. Chronic infection with HAV is not seen.

The clinical picture varies with age, more severe disease being seen in adults and mainly asymptomatic infections in young children. The disease is usually self-limiting although protracted. About half of the clinical cases of hepatitis in industrialized countries is caused by HAV with considerable costs for society. Mortality due to liver damage can occur in adults. In developing countries the disease is usually acquired in early childhood giving little or no clinical manifestations. Over 90 % of adults in these countries have antibodies to the virus and life-long immunity to the disease. With rising hygienic standard and sanitation, the situation in industrialized countries has rapidly changed towards low rates of antibody among adults [92]. Gamma globulin can prevent clinical infection but the protection is of short duration. Prevention by vaccination represents therefore a preferable approach.

The two classical approaches to vaccine development, killed (inactivated) virus vaccines and attenuated, live vaccines are currently explored. The first experimental killed vaccine was prepared from marmoset liver as early as 1978 by Provost and coworkers. This formaldehyde-inactivated vaccine was found to be immunogenic in monkeys and protective against virus challenge. The study proved the feasibility of the approach and was pursued with virus propagated in cell culture when this technique became available. The same group later developed a formaldehyde-inactivated vaccine from virus grown in tissue culture with equally encouraging results in experimental studies [93].

Several other inactivated HAV vaccines have been developed [94, 96]. A recent study demonstrated the safety and immunogenicity of a formaldehyde-killed HAV vaccine from virus solely propagated in human diploid fibroblasts [92]. Three doses of the vaccine were administered to half of the subjects as plain vaccine and half of the subjects received an alum-adsorbed preparation. The alum-adsorbed preparation was more immunogenic and induced neutralizing antibodies in all the volunteers.

Attenuated, live HAV vaccines have also been developed by several groups [96, 99]. Attenuation of the virus strain was assessed in animal models. A recent clinical study in seronegative adult volunteers with an attenuated strain confirmed the animal safety and immunogenicity data [100]. A seroconversion was noted in all subjects and no adverse reactions, neither in the form of clinical symptoms nor pathological laboratory tests (liver enzymes), were noted. The virus was excreted in low concentrations, as previously noted in experimental studies.

The encouraging results in both development lines indicate that a vaccine against HAV can be expected to be available in the near future. Whether both types of vaccines are going to be used remains an open issue. A disadvantage of the killed vaccine as compared to a live, attenuated vaccine could be a possibly shorter duration of immunity. This theoretical draw-back of a killed vaccine may however outweigh the safety considerations that have to be applied to a live vaccine. The balance of safe attenuation and retained immunogenicity is difficult. In addition, the risk for a reversion to a wild virus state has always to be kept in mind in analogy with polio virus, another member of the picornavirus group.

3.17 Rotavirus Vaccine

Rotavirus, a member of the *reovirus* group, was first identified as the cause of gastroenteritis by Bishop and coworkers [101] and Flewett and coworkers [102] in 1973. Reovirus as cause of diarrhea in animals has been known for many years but in human disease the first observations were made by electron microscopy. The virus was later shown to grow in tissue culture but has a fastidious growth pattern in comparison to animal reoviruses. The virus is transmitted by the oral-fecal route. The disease is characterized by watery diarrhea, often in conjunction with vomiting and fever. The resulting dehydration is the cause of the severe clinical picture requiring hospitalization in a large proportion of cases and of death in developing countries.

Rotavirus diarrhea is predominantly a disease of young children but adults can also be affected. Peak incidence rates in industrialized countries occur during the winter months in children 6-24 months of age. In developing countries with tropical climate, the seasonal variation is not pronounced and many cases are seen in infants under 6 months of age. In industrialized countries, approximately 60 % of diarrheal disease requiring hospitalization is caused by rotavirus. In developing countries, rotavirus has been estimated to cause 30 % of diarrhea - associated mortality in children 6-23 months of age, resulting in 500 000 - 1 000 000 deaths per year.

The capsid of rotavirus consists of two layers. The inner capsid contains a group antigen, VP6, common to human and animal group A rotaviruses. The outer capsid contains two major antigens, VP7 and VP4, both involved in virus neutralization. Based on differences in VP7, four human serotypes, 1-4, are currently recognized although virus isolates not belonging to any of those types have recently been described. Epidemiologic studies have shown type 1 to be the dominating serotype, especially in the winter infections of temperate climates. The remaining serotypes, types 3, 2 and 4 give more sporadic infections in the given order. Types 2 and 3 seem to be more common in tropical climates. Neutralizing antibodies developing after natural disease are mainly serotype-specific although some heterologous neutralization seems to be induced by a surface group epitope located on VP3.

Protection by animal rotavirus against human rotavirus has been shown and represents the rationale behind the development of bovine and simian rotavirus as vaccine candidate for live, oral rotavirus vaccines. Two bovine strains, RIT 4236 and WC3, have been tested in clinical trials in humans. RIT 4237, the most extensively investigated strain, showed 50-60 % protection against diarrhea of any severity and 80-90 % against severe disease in children 6-12 months of age receiving one or two doses of vaccine in two trials in Finland [103, 104]. In a study in Rwanda, however, one dose of the vaccine to 3-8 months old infants conferred no immunity against any forms of the disease [105]. Studies in Gambia and in Peru showed 30-40 % protective efficacy with three doses [106, 107]. Due to the encountered difficulties in developing countries, the vaccine has been withdrawn from clinical trials by the manufacturer.

Another bovine strain, WC3, evaluated in Philadelphia, was found to confer 76 % protection against all diarrheal diseases and 100 % against moderate-severe disease during a mainly serotype 1 rotavirus season [108]. The vaccine is currently undergoing clinical evaluation in different parts of the world. Both bovine rotavirus vaccines have been found to be essentially without side effects.

Rhesus monkey rotavirus, RRV-1 strain, is the other extensively investigated rotavirus vaccine. High dose of the virus (10^5 plaque forming units) in a study in Sweden gave 48 % protection against rotavirus diarrhea of any severity and 80 % for clinically significant episodes in children 4-12 months of age [109]. At this dosage, however, the vaccine induced considerable side effects. A lower dose of 10^4 plaque forming units has been used in subsequent trials. The best results, 68 % protection against rotavirus diarrhea of any severity and 100 % against severe disease, were obtained in a study in Venezuela against rotavirus infection caused mainly by serotype 3, of the same serotpye as the vaccine strain [110]. Three studies in the US and one in Finland showed much lower protective efficacy, ranging from 0-38 % for rotavirus diarrhea of any severity and 0-67 % for severe disease [111]. Even the lower dosage gave rise to significant side effects.

Reassorted viruses represent a new approach to the rotavirus vaccine problem. The human rotavirus gene coding for VP7 is preserved while animal viruses, rhesus or bovine, donate genes coding for growth and attenuation. Several reassorted virus vaccines are currently undergoing clinical trials. One of them is W1 79-9, a reassortant between the bovine vaccine strain WC3 and a human serotype 1 rotavirus. VP7 reassorted bovine viruses for serotypes 1-4 have been produced as have reassortants for human VP7 serotypes 1, 2 and 4 with rhesus rotavirus strains. Safety and immunogenicity trials with all these vaccines alone and in combination have just been completed or are under way [112]. Preliminary data on protection seem promising.

Reassortants with natural attenuation, so-called "nursery strains" have been isolated from asymptomatic infants. One such strain, M37, has serotype specificity for both type 1 (on VP7) and for type 4 (on VP3). This strain is also subject to clinical trials in humans.

In summary, the completed clinical trials indicate that sufficient heterotypic immunity is not induced by a vaccine containing only one serotype. Use of multivalent vaccine of single VP7 gene reassortants might solve the problem but it is not yet known whether VP7 alone is sufficient for protection and whether interference between the strains will occur. Interference with oral polio vaccine has been noted in some trials of animal rotavirus vaccine and may be a practical problem for the second generation of rotavirus vaccines as well. A vaccine against rotavirus infection will no doubt be developed but the task seems more difficult than indicated by the first encouraging results.

3.18 Respiratory Syncytial Virus Vaccine

Respiratory syncytial virus (RSV) is an RNA virus belonging to the *paramyxovirus* group. RSV is the leading cause of bronchiolitis and pneumonia in young infants and accounts for the majority of hospitalizations in this age group. Reinfections, also in adults, occur frequently but the primary infection is generally the most severe. The disease is one of the most important diseases in children and prevention by immunization is a major goal of vaccine development [113].

The development of an RSV vaccine is associated with numerous problems. The peak incidence of severe disease in young infants necessitates very early immunization in the presence of maternal antibody. The occurrence of at least two subtypes recognized only in recent years has important implications for the pathology of the disease and for vaccine research. The failure of a formaldehyde-inactivated RSV vaccine in the 1960s had a tremendous impact on the field, appreciable till the present days.

Immunization of infants with this formalin-inactivated vaccine led to typical but severe disease upon exposure to wild-type virus. The vaccine elicited an antibody response of non-functional antibodies that was comparable to that seen after natural disease. Neutralizing antibodies to the major protective antigens, the surface F and G glycoprotein, were however not elicited or were much lower than after natural infection. In particular, the functional antibodies that inhibit syncytia formation – fusion-inhibiting (F1) antibodies – were lacking [114].

The development of a cotton rat model for experimental studies on the disease-enhancement by this vaccine has given important information on the pathology of this reaction [115]. It was shown that the large amounts of non-functional antibodies elicited by the formalin-inactivated vaccine led to antigen-antibody complex formation in the lung of the animals upon intranasal wild-virus challenge. The model has great importance for the experimental evaluation of future vaccines for the risk of potentiation of disease.

Since the failure of the formalin-inactivated RSV vaccine had many features in common with the corresponding failure with measles virus, the alternative approach of live, attenuated vaccine as for measles has been extensively investigated. Temperature-sensitive mutants were developed and tested in humans in the early 1970s. This vaccine was not protective and the vaccine strain recovered from volunteers showed an altered temperature sensitivity intermediate between vaccine and wild strains [116]. Efforts to develop attenuated vaccines continued with equally disappointing results [117].

New temperature sensitive mutants are still being tested in humans [118]. Even if stable mutants can be produced, it remains unclear whether a live vaccine for RSV represents a realistic alternative. Presence of neutralizing maternal antibodies has been a problem also for early immunization against measles. RSV vaccine will have to be administered at an even earlier age for protection against the severe primary infection of infants.

Subunit vaccines represent a currently pursued alternative [119]. Expression of the G and F glycoproteins in vaccinia virus has shown both antigens to elicit high levels of neutralizing antibodies and protection in different animal models. The F protein has been found to be a more important protective antigen than the G protein. A subunit vaccine based on purified F glycoprotein is currently tested in adults and toddlers with promising results. The prospect for a vaccine against RSV seems therefore more promising at present than for many years.

3.19 Parainfluenza Vaccine

Parainfluenza viruses (PIV) belong to the *paramyxovirus* group. Four types are identified and PIV 1-3 cause severe respiratory infections in infants. Next after RSV, PIV-3 is the most common cause of bronchiolitis and pneumonia in young children. PIV-1 and PIV-2 are primarily associated with croup. The peak age incidence for PIV infections is in older infants than that for RSV infection [113]. The major protective antigens of parainfluenza viruses are the hemagglutinin-neuraminidase (HN) and fusion (F) glycoproteins, each separately capable of inducing protection in animal models. Only one type of PIV is recognized for each serotype, with evidence of conservation of neutralizing epitopes.

Current vaccine development includes development of subunit vaccines based on the HN and F glycoproteins and expression of these antigens in vaccinia and *baculoviruses* [120]. Numerous experimental studies with both approaches have shown promising results. These inactivated vaccines can be tested in the cotton rat model for safety regarding disease enhancement since formalin-inactivated PIV gives rise to disease-potentiation in this model in analogy with RSV.

Live PIV vaccine has been developed by two distinct approaches [120]. One vaccine is based on temperature-sensitive mutants of PIV-3. Such cold-adapted mutants have been found effective and stable in animal models and are ready for clinical trials in humans. The other live PIV-3 vaccine is a bovine strain of PIV-3. This vaccine has shown promising results in experimental models as well and is advancing towards clinical trials. An effective PIV vaccine, either attenuated or subunit, seems to be a feasible goal within the near future.

3.20 Dengue Fever Vaccine

Dengue virus belongs to the *togavirus* group and is transmitted by (*Aedes*) mosquitoes [76, 77]. As for the closely related Japanese encephalitis, the range of human disease goes from subclinical infection to a debilitating, febrile disease to a severe hemorrhagic fever/shock syndrome with high fatality rate. These clinical manifestations can be caused by any of the four serotypes, 1-4. The serotypes are antigenically related but not cross-protective. Dengue virus has some common epitopes with other *flaviviruses* with cross-neutralizing antibodies and probably some short term immunity induced by Japanese encephalitis virus vaccine [84]. Dengue disease is increasing in the tropical parts of the world.

In spite of more than 40 years of efforts, vaccine development has been unsuccessful. Virus production in tissue culture being limited, development of killed vaccine has not been pursued. Live, attenuated dengue vaccines against all four types have been produced. The strains were however either over-attenuated and lost immunogenicity or caused dengue disease in volunteers. More reliable markers for attenuation are therefore being investigated [121].

A major cause for concern has been the general view that the hemorrhagic fever/shock syndrome would be mainly seen in individuals with previous antibody to other serotypes. Vaccine development would therefore have to be made in parallel for all four serotypes. The evidence for this association has recently been questioned [122].

The most encouraging results with attenuated vaccines have recently been reported for a dengue 2 virus strain not causing clinical disease but inducing immune response in humans [123]. The other line of development is the identification of protective proteins. The virus-specific nonstructural polypeptide NS 1 and envelope glycoprotein (E) represent such candidates. Epitopes inducing protective but not infection-enhancing antibodies on these proteins are being investigated. Variable results regarding immunogenicity and protection in different animal models have been obtained [124, 125].

3.21 Herpes simplex Vaccine

Herpes simplex viruses (HSV) are members of the *herpes-virus* group. Two types are recognized, HSV-1 and HSV-2 causing labial and genital infections respectively. Primary infection with HSV-1 occurs in childhood while HSV-2 is acquired at sexual debut. Both viruses establish latency with recurrent clinical manifestations experienced by approximately one-third of humanity. Central nervous involvement in HSV-1 infection is a severe encephalitis. The corresponding manifestation with HSV-2 is a milder meningitis, seen in 10-30 % of recurrent HSV-2 infections. HSV can transform cells *in vitro*. The possible association of HSV-2 with cervix carcinoma makes vaccine development an even more challenging but difficult task.

Crude surface antigen preparations have been evaluated in animal models. Some studies indicated protection against lethal challenge in animals but none showed protection against establishement of latency [126]. In humans, some studies found an effect by diminsihed frequency and severity of recurrent episodes but none of the studies were blinded and controlled. Purified protective antigens, gB, gC, gD, gE and gH have been used alone or in combinations. Several experimental systems showed good immunogenicity and protection against challenge but none protected against latency. Similarly, these antigens expressed in vaccinia virus showed promising results against acute infection but not against latent infection in animal models.

Live vaccines in the form of genetically engineered deletion mutants have also been extensively investigated. A mutant was found to be protective against challenge with both HSV types in non-human primates. Immunization did however not prevent establishment of latency. Also, the possibility of recombinants between the genetic mutant and wild-strains *in vivo* is a disquieting possibility to be kept in mind.

3.22 Cytomegalovirus Vaccine

Cytomegalovirus (CMV) is a member of the *herpes virus* group. The primary CMV infection is in a vast majority of cases an asymptomatic infection, usually in childhood. Clinical manifestation is mainly a febrile disease with unspecific symptoms but occasionally, the clinical picture mimics infectious mononucleosis. After primary infection, the virus remains latent in the body but causes usually no symptoms. In patients immune-compromised by disease or therapy, CMV is not a benign virus. These patients can suffer severe infections with high mortality rate, especially after primary infection. Also the relative immunesuppression of pregnancy can cause reactivation of the virus with consequent infection of the fetus. Primary infection in the mother during pregnancy results usually in the most severe manifestations of congenital disease. Congenital CMV is now the leading congenital infection, estimated to affect 0,2-2,5 % of all live births. Symptomatic infection is seen in only 5-10 % at birth but 5-20 % of the originally asymptomatic children develop late manifestations.

Development of live virus vaccine was started in the 1970s in spite of the possible oncogenic potential of the virus [127]. The most extensively studied Towne vaccine strain has been found to be immunogenic, non-reactogenic, was not excreted following immunization and doesn't seem to give rise to latent infection. Studies in renal transplant recipients demonstrated that immunization protected from severe CMV infection. A recent challenge study in volunteers with the wildtype Toledo strain demonstrated a dose-dependent protection [128]. The encouraging results in renal transplant patients indicate that the vaccine could be of value for CMV-negative recipients. Immunizations of millions of healthy adolescent girls for prevention of congenital CMV might seem less attractive with a live CMV vaccine.

Development of subunit vaccine is also being pursued but knowledge of protective antigens for CMV is more limited than for herpes simplex virus. A major envelope protein complex consisting of a 130 kD and a 58 kD species has been shown to induce neutralizing antibodies and a cellular immune response in experimental animals. This protein complex has also been expressed in vaccinia virus and induced neutralizing antibodies in animals. Other studies have investigated a single glycoprotein of 86 kD that was shown also to induce neutralizing antibodies.

3.23 Human Immunodeficiency Virus Vaccine

Human immunodeficiency viruses (HIV) are RNA viruses belonging to the *retrovirus* group. HIV-1 was isolated from patients with acquired immunodeficiency syndrome (AIDS) in 1983 by Montagnier and coworkers and in 1984 by Gallo and coworkers and Levy and coworkers. Another virus causing similar clinical disease in West Africa was isolated and termed HIV-2 in 1985. A virus causing immunodeficiency in monkeys was simultaneously demonstrated and named simian immunodeficiency virus (SIV).

Transmission of the disease is mainly sexual but also by blood and blood products. In certain parts of the world, HIV infection is the most common congenital/perinatal infection in newborns. Infectivity approaches 100 % but in a few instances, infected individuals are known to have escaped disease. Viral infection is followed by an asymptomatic period, usually lasting months or sometimes years. The first clinical symptoms in some individuals are unspecific, influenza-like with swollen lymph nodes lasting a few days or weeks. After a variable asymptomatic period signs of progressive immunesuppression become manifest with increasing susceptibility to other microbial infections and sometimes cancer, Kaposi sarcoma.

Vaccine development against HIV is complicated by practically all the difficulties encountered separately with other viral vaccines and it has some additional problems caused by the nature of the disease [129, 130]. The problems encountered with other viruses causing latent infections such as herpes-viruses have been discussed (see herpes simplex and cytomegalovirus vaccines). The high degree of genetic variation in the genome of HIV isolates represents an influenza A vaccine type of problem where the antigenic drift has led to only partial protection by even multivalent vaccines (see influenza A vaccine). The lack of a good animal model represents a major problem and the scarcity of the best test animal at present, the chimpanzee, renders research more difficult. Recent reports of the possibility of using rabbits as experimental animal might represent a solution. The ethical and legal considerations that accompanies even Phase 1 and 2 for testing of immunogenicity and safety in humans are considerable. Phase 3 clinical trials for demonstration of efficacy can be difficult to conduct for the same considerations. In spite of all the difficulties, considerable effort is directed to the development of a HIV vaccine.

The primary target cell of the virus is the lymphocyte but also macrophages can be infected. The receptor on lymphocytes, CD4, represents a first target for vaccine development and studies with anti-idiotype antibodies are currently under way. Major HIV-1 gene products investigated as potential immunogens in a vaccine against HIV are the gp160 envelope glycoprotein composed of gp120 and gp41 (encoded by the env gene), p55, p24, p18 and p15 (gag gene) and p64, p53 and p31 (pol gene). Vaccines based on gp160 protein are currently tested in humans [130, 131]. gp160 is either administered as purified protein or by use of live vaccinia virus used as expression vector. Vaccinia virus expressing gp120 and gp41 are also currently being tested in humans. Studies in chimpanzees with these vaccine candidates have generally been disappointing with regard to immunogenicity and protection but some human data with the vaccinia virus approach have shown that good and long lasting immune response can be obtained.

Killed whole virus vaccine for post exposure treatment was suggested by Salk [131]. Concerns were raised due to presence of genetic material and for risk of potentiation. Studies in monkeys showed, however, that immunization of previously infected chimpanzees resulted in the disappearance of cultivable virus. Studies in patients with AIDS-related complex, an early stage of AIDS, showed no ill effects and vaccination seemed to have improved the cell-mediated immune response of the vaccinees.

3.24 References

1. Mitchell, C. D. and Balfour, H. H., Jr., *Prog. Med. Virol.* (1985), **31**, 1-42.
2. Markowitz, L. E. and Bernier, R. H., *Pediatr. Infect. Dis. J.* (1987), **6**, 809-812.
3. WHO Expert Committee on Biological Standardization, *WHO Tech. Tep. Ser.* (1966), **329**.
4. WHO Expert Committee on Biological Standardization, *WHO Tech. Rep. Ser.* (1982), **673**.
5. Centers for Disease Control, *MMWR* (1987), **36**, 301-305.

5a. *MMWR* (1989), **38**, 5-9.

5b. *Pediatrics* (1989), **84**, 1110-1113.

6. Bart, K. J., Orenstein, W. A. and Hinman, A. R., *Dev. Biol. Stand.* (1986), **65**, 45-52.
7. Norrby, E., Enders-Ruckle, G. and ter Meulen, V., *J. Infect. Dis.* (1975), **132**, 262-269.
8. Varsanyi, T. M., Morein, B., Löve, A. and Norrby, E., *J. Virol.* (1987), **61**, 3896-3901.
9. Hilleman, M. R., *In:* Modern Trends in Medical Virology, **vol. 2,** Butterworths, London (1970), 241-261.
10. Penttinen, K., Cantell, K., Somer, P. and Poikolainen, A., *Am. J. Epidemiol.* (1968), **88**, 234-244.
11. Hilleman, M. R., Weibel, R. E., Buynak, E. B., Stokes, J., Jr., et al., *N. Engl. J. Med.* (1967), **276**, 252-258.
12. Centers for Disease Control, *MMWR* (1983),**32**, 391-398.
13. Andre, F. E. and Peetermans, J., *Dev. Biol. Stand.* (1986), **65**, 101-107.
14. Glück, R., Hoskins, J. M., Wegmann, A., Just, M., et al., *Dev. Biol. Stand.* (1986), **65**, 29-35.
15. WHO Expert Committee on biological standardizing, *WHO Tech. Rep. Ser.* (1987), **760.**
16. Recommendation of the Immunization Practices Advisory Committee (ACIP), *MMWR* (1982), **31**, 617-625.
17. Penttinen, K., Helle, E. P. and Norrby, E., *Dev. Biol. Stand.* (1979), **43**, 265-268.

17a. *Lancet* (1989), **ii**, 394.

18. Löve, A., Rydbeck, R., Utter, G., Örvell, C., et al., *J. Virol.* (1986), **58,** 220-222.
19. Perkins, F. T., *Rev. Infect. Dis.* (1985), **7, Suppl. 1,** 73-76.
20. Plotkin, S. A. and Buser, F., *Rev. Infect. Dis.* (1985), **7, Suppl. 1**, 77-78.
21. WHO Expert Committee on Biological Standardization, *WHO Tech. Rep. Ser.* (1977), **610.**
22. WHO Expert Committee on Biological Standardization, *WHO Tech. Rep. Ser.* (1981), **658.**
23. Dudgeon, J. A., *Rev. Infect. Dis.* (1985), **7**, 185-190.
24. Recommendation of the Immunization Practices Advisory Committee (ACIP), *MMWR* (1984), **33**, 301-318.
25. Christenson, B., Böttiger, M. and Heller, L., *Br. Med. J.* (1983), **287**, 389-391.
26. Centers for Disease Control, *MMWR* (1987), **36**, 457-461.
27. Recommendation of the Immunization Practices Advisory Committee (ACIP), *MMWR* (1986), **35**, 577-579.
28. Deforest, A., Long, S. S., Lischner, H. W., Girone, J. A. C., et al., *Pediatrics* (1988), **81**, 237-246.
29. Peltola, H. and Heinonen, O. P., *Lancet* (1986), **i,** 939-942.
30. Arbeter, A. M., Baker, L., Starr, S. E. and Plotkin, S. A., *Dev. Biol. Stand.* (1986), **65**, 89-93.
31. Schonberger, L. B., Kaplan, J., Kim-Farley, R., Moore, M. et al, *Rev. Infect. Dis.* (1984), **6, Suppl. 2**, 424-426.
32. Salk, J., *Pediatr. Infect. Dis. J.* (1987), **6**, 889-893.
33. Wilson, G. S., The hazards of immunization. University of London, The Athlone Press, (1967).
34. Sabin, A. B., *J. Infect. Dis.* (1985), **151**, 420-436.
35. Sabin, A. B., *Pediatr. Infect. Dis. J.* (1987), **6**, 887-889.
36. Böttiger, M., *Dev. Biol. Stand.* (1981), **47**, 227-232.
37. Lapinleimu, K. and Stenvik, M., *Dev. Biol. Stand* (1981), **47**, 241-246.

38. Bijkerk, H., *Dev. Biol. Stand* (1981), **47**, 233-240.
39. WHO Expert Committee on Biological Standardization, *WHO Tech. Rep. Ser.* (1983), **687**.
40. McBean, A. M., and Modlin, J. F., *Pediatr. Infect. Dis. J.* (1987), **6**, 881-887.
41. Lapinleimu, K., *In:* Proceedings of the 11th Symposium of the European Association Against Poliomyelitis and Allied Diseases, Rome 1966, Brussels European Association Against Poliomyelitis, (1967), 119-125.
42. van Wezel, A. L., van Steenis, G., Hannik, C. A. and Cohen, H., *Dev. Biol. Stand* (1987), **41**, 159-168.
43. Robertson, S. E., Traverso, H. P., Drucker, J. A., Rovira, E. Z., et al., *Lancet* (1988), **i**, 897-899.
44. Montagnon, B. J., Fanget, B., Nicolas, A. J., *Dev. Biol. Stand.* (1981), **47**, 55-64.
45. WHO Expert Committee on Biological Standardization, *WHO Tech. Rep. Ser.* (1987), **745**.
46. Prevention of liver cancer, *WHO Tech. Tep. Ser.* (1983), **691**.
47. McLean, A. A., *Rev. Infect. Dis.* (1986), **8**, 591-598.
48. Szmuness, W., Stevens, C. E., Harley, E. J., Zang, E. A., et al., *N. Engl. J. Med.* (1980), **303**, 833-841.
49. WHO Expert Committee on Biological Standardization, *WHO Tech. Tep. Ser.* (1985), **725**.
50. Recommendation of the Immunization Practices Advisory Committee (ACIP), *MMWR.* (1985), **34**, 313-335.
51. Recommendation of the Immunization Practices Advisory Committee (ACIP), *MMWR.* (1987), **36**, 353-366.
52. Eder, G., McDonel, J. L. and Dorner, F., *In:* Progress in Liver Diseases, **vol. 8**, Grune and Stratton, New York (1986), 367-394.
53. Zuckerman, A., *Vaccine* (1987), **5**, 165-167.
54. Standring, D. N. and Rutter, W. J., *In:* Progress in Liver Diseases, **vol. 8**, Grune and Stratton, New York (1986), 331-333.
55. WHO Expert Committee on Rabies, *WHO Tech. Rep. Ser.* (1984), **709.**
56. Centers for Disease Control, *MMWR* (1986), **35**, 430-432.
57. Sureau, P., *Adv. Biochem. Eng. Biotechnol.* (1987), **34**, 111-128.
58. Perry, B. D., *Vet. Clin. North. Am. Small Anim. Pract.* (1987), **17**, 73-89.
59. Wilde, H., Chomchey, P., Prakongsri, S. and Punyaratabandhu, P., *Lancet* (1987), **ii**, 1275.
60. Centers for Disease Control, *MMWR* (1987), **36**, 759-765.
61. Centers for Disease Control, *MMWR* (1984), **33**, 185-187.
62. Swanson, M. C., Rosanoff, E., Gurwith, M., Deitch, M., et al., *J. Infect. Dis.* (1987), **155**, 909-913.
63. Grantström, M., Eriksson, M. and Edevåg, G., *J. Biol. Stand.* (1987), **15**, 193-197.
64. Morein, B. and Simons, K., *Vaccine* (1985), **3**, 83-93.
65. Stuart-Harris, C. H. and Schild, G. C., Influenza, The Viruses and Disease, E. Arnold Ltd., London (1976).
66. Wright, P. F. and Karzon, D. T., *Prog. Med. Virol.* (1987), **34**, 70-88.
67. WHO Expert Committee on Biological Standardization, *WHO Tech. Rep. Ser.* (1979), **638.**
68. Recommendations of the Immunization Practices Advisory Committee (ACIP), *MMWR* (1987), **36,** 373-387.
69. Gross, P. A., Gould, A. L. and Brown, A. E., *Rev. Infect. Dis.* (1985), **7**, 613-618.
70. Strassburg, M. A., Greenland, S., Sorvillo, F. J., Lieb, L. E., et al., *Vaccine* (1986), **4**, 38-44.
71. Ostrove, J. M. and Inchauspé, G., *Ann. Intern. Med.* (1988), **108**, 221-227.
72. Takahashi, M., *Pediatrics* (1986), **78, suppl.**, 736-741.
73. Weibel, R. E., Neff, B. J., Kuter, B. J., Guess, H. A., et al., *N. Engl. J. Med.* (1984), **310**, 1409-1415.
74. Gershon, A. A., Steinberg, S. P., Gelb, L., and The National Institute of Allergy and Infectious Diseases Varicella Vaccine Collaborative Study Group, *Pediatrics* (1986), **78**, **suppl.**, 757-762.
75. Arthropod-borne and rodent-borne viral diseases, *WHO Techn. Rep. Ser.* (1985), **719.**
76. Viral haemorrhagic fevers, *WHO Tech. Rep. Ser.* (1985), **721.**
77. Smithburn, K. C., Cureiux, C., Koerber, R., Penna, H. A., et al., Yellow Fever Vaccination, World Health Organization, Geneva, (1956).

78. Roche, J. C., Jouan, A., Brisou, B., Rodhain, R., et al., *Vaccine* (1986), **4**, 163-165.
79. WHO Expert Committee on Biological Standardization, *WHO Tech. Rep. Ser.* (1976), **594.**
80. Smordodintsev, A. A., Dubov, A. V., Ilyenko, V. I. and Platonov, V. G., *J. Hyg.* (1969), **67**, 13-20.
81. Kuntz, C., Heinz, F. X., and Hofmann, H., *J. Med. Virol.* (1980), **6**, 103-109.
82. Oya, A., *In:* The vaccination. Theory and practice, Fukumi, H. (ed.), International Medical Foundation of Japan, (1975), 69-82.
83. WHO Expert Committee on Biological Standardization, *WHO Tech. Rep. Ser.* (1966), **323.**
84. Hoke, C. H., Nisalak, A., Sangawhipa, N., Jatanasen, S., Laorakapongse, T., et al., *New Engl. J. Med.* (1988), **319**, 608-614.
85. Recommendation of the Immunization Practices Advisory Committee (ACIP), (1985), **34**, 341-342.
86. Meiklejohn, G., *J. Infect. Dis.* (1983), **148**, 775-784.
87. Takafuji, E. T., Gaydos, J. C., Allen, R. G. and Top, F. H., Jr., *J. Infect. Dis.* (1979), **140**, 48-53.
88. Randall, R., Binn, L. N. and Harrison, V. R., *J. Immunol.* (1964), **93**, 293-299.
89. Niklasson, B., *Scand. J. Infect. Dis.* (1982), **14**, 105-109.
90. Feinstone, S. M., Kapikian, A. Z. and Purcell, R. H., *Science* (1973), **182**, 1026-1028.
91. Provost, P. J. and Hillerman, M. R., *Proc. Soc. Exp. Biol. Med.* (1979), **160**, 213-221.
92. Flehmig, B., Heinricy, U. and Pfisterer, M., *Lancet* (1989), **i**, 1039-1041.
93. Provost, P. J., Hughes, J. V., Miller, W. J., Glesa, P. A., et al., *J. Med. Virol.* (1986), **19**, 23-31.
94. Binn, L. N., Bancroft, W. H., Eckels, K. H., Marchwicki, R. H., et al., *In:* Viral hepatitis and liver disease, Zuckerman, A. (ed.), New York Alan R. Liss Inc., (1988), 91-93.
95. Sjogren, M. H., Eckels, K. H., Binn, L. N., Dubois, D. R., et al., *In:* Viral hepatitis and liver disease, Zuckerman, A. (ed.), New York Alan R. Liss Inc., (1988), 94-96.
96. Chaudhary, R. K., Parker, C. and Mo, T., *In:* Viral hepatitis and liver diseases, Zuckerman, A. (ed.), New York Alan R. Liss Inc., (1988), 97-99.
97. Flehmig, B., Mauler, R. F., Noll, G., Weinmann, E., et al., *In:* Viral hepatitis and liver disease, Zuckerman, A. (ed.), New York Alan R. Liss Inc, (1988), 87-90.
98. Feinstone, S. M., Daemer, R. J., Gust, I. D. and Purcell, R. H., *Develop. Biol. Standard* (1983), **54**, 429-432.
99. Hu, M., Scheid, R., Deinhardt, F., Gauss-Müller, V., et al., *In:* Viral hepatitis and liver diseases, Zuckerman, A. (ed.), New York Alan R. Liss Inc., (1988), 81-82.
100. Mao, J. S., Dong, D. X., Zhang, H. Y., Chen, N. L., et al., *J. Infect. Dis.* (1989), **159** , 621-624.
101. Bishop, R. F., Davidson, G. P., Holmes, I. H. and Ruck, B. J., *Lancet* (1973), **ii**, 1281-1283.
102. Flewett, T. H., Bryden, A. S. and Davies, H., *Lancet* (1973), **ii**, 1497.
103. Vesikari, T., Isolauri, A., d'Hondt, E., Delem, A., *Lancet* (1984), **i**, 977-981.
104. Vesikari, T., Isolauri, E., Delem, A., d'Hondt, E., *J. Pediadr.* (1985), **107**, 189-194.
105. de Mol, P., Zissis, G., Butzler, J.-P., Mutwewingabo, A., *Lancet* (1986), **ii**, 108.
106. Hanlon, P., Hanlon, L., Marsch, V., Byass, P., *Lancet* (1987), **i**, 1342-1345.
107. Lanata, C. F., Black, R. E., del Aguila, R., Gil, A., et al., *J. Infect. Dis.* (1989), **159**, 452-459.
108. Clark, H. F., Borian, F. E., Bell, L. M., Modesto, K., et al., *J. Infect. Dis.* (1988), **158**, 570-587.
109. Gothefors, L., Wadell, G., Juto, P., Taniguchi, K., et al., *J. Infect. Dis.* (1989), **159**, 753-757.
110. Flores, J., Perez-Schael, I., Gonzalez, M., Garcia, D., et al., *Lancet* (1987), **i**, 882-884.
111. Christy, C., Madore, H. P., Pichichero, M. E., Gala, C., et al., *Pediatr. Infect. Dis. J.* (1988), **7**, 645-650.
112. Halsey, N. A., Anderson, E. L., Sears, S. D., Steinhoff, M., et al., *J. Infect. Dis.* (1988), **158**, 1261-1267.
113. Murphy, B. R., Prince, G. A., Collins, P. L., van Wyke, K., Coelingh, et al., *Virus Res.* (1988), **11**, 1-15.
114. Murphy, B. R. and Walsh, E. E., *J. Clin. Microbiol.* (1988), **26**, 1595-1597.
115. Prince, G. A., Jensen, A. B., Hemming, V. G., Murphy, B. R., et al., *J. Virol.* (1986), **57**, 721-728.
116. Hodes, D. S., Wha, H. K., Parrott, R. H., Camargo, E., et al., *Proc. Soc. Exp. Biol. Med.* (1974), **145**, 1158-1164.
117. Belshe, R. B., van Voris, L. P. and Mufson, M. A., *J. Infect. Dis.* (1982), **145**, 311-319.
118. McKay, E., Higgins, P., Tyrell, D. and Pringle, C., *J. Med. Virol.* (1988), **25**, 411-421.

119. Pringle, C. R., *Bull WHO* (1987), **65**, 133-137.
120. Murphy, B. R., *Bull WHO* (1988), **66**, 391-397.
121. Innis, B. L., Eckels, K. H., Kraiselburd, E., Dubois, D. R., *J. Infect. Dis.* (1988), **158**, 876-880.
122. Rosen, L., *J. Infect. Dis.* (1989), **II, suppl. 4**, S840-S842.
123. Shamarapravati, N., Yoksan, S., Chayaniyayothin, T., Angsubphakorn, S., et al., *Bull WHO* (1987), **65**, 189-195.
124. Bray, M., Zhao, B., Markoff, L., Eckels, K. H., *J. Virol.* (1989), **63**, 2853-2856.
125. Eubel, V., Kinney, R. M., Esposito, J. J., Cropp, C. B., *J. Gen. Virol.* (1988), **69**, 1921-1929.
126. Dix, R. D., *In: Prog. Med. Virol.* (1987), **34**, 89-128, J. L. Melnick, (ed.), Karger, Basel.
127. Farrar, G. H., Bull, J. R. and Greenaway, P. J., et al., *Vaccine* (1986), **4**, 217-224.
128. Plotkin, S. A., Starr, S. E., Friedman, H. M., Gönczöl, E., *J. Infect. Dis.* (1989), **159**, 860-865.
129. Katzenstein, D. A., Swyer, L. A., and Quinnan, G. V., Jr., *AIDS* (1988), **2**, 151-155.
130. Koff, W. C. and Hotz, D. F., *Science* (1988), **241**, 426-432.
131. Snart, R. S., *AIDS* (1988), **2, suppl.,** S107-S111.

4. Vaccines Against Parasites

4.1 Vaccines Against Helminthiasis

S. J. Cryz, Jr.

4.1.1 Introduction

Helminthic diseases are endemic in most sub-tropical and tropical areas of the world and are caused by a number of related parasites (Tab. 4-1). Due to difficulties in disease reporting within the areas, it is impossible to accurately determine the number of individuals infected. However, broad worldwide estimates have been made for schistosomiasis (300 million) [1] and filariasis (200 million) [2]. One can therefore presume that somewhere in the region of 750 million to 1 billion people are suffering from some type of helminth infection. Since certain of these diseases are of a chronic debilitating nature, the health care costs and economic losses are staggering. Although substantial advances have been made in the chemotherapy of helminth diseases, treatment in most cases is protracted and not always successful.

Tab. 4-1 Helminth pathogens of humans and animals.

Disease	Etiological agents
Schistosomiasis	*Schistosoma haematobium* *S. mansoni* *S. japonicum*
Gastrointestinal nematodes	*Ascaris* spp. *Trichinella* spp. *Strongyloides* spp. *Ancylostoma* spp. *Necator* spp.
Filariasis	*Wucheria bancrofti* *Brugia malayi* *Onchocerca volvulus*
Cestodiasis	*Echinococcus granulosus* *E. multilocularis* *Taenia solium*

Unfortunately, progress towards the development of vaccines to prevent helminth diseases has lagged appreciably behind strides made in chemotherapy. To date, the only successes in this area have been vaccines for domestic animals. A great deal of the problem is that the host-parasite relationship has evolved to the point were the immune response mounted by the host is insufficient to eradicate the invading pathogen. However, recent advances in understanding the anti-parasitic immune response has provided new insight as to the protective elements of such a response. Coupled with the use of recombinant DNA technology to produce purified parasite antigens, the time where effective anti-helminth vaccines become available may not be far off.

4.1.2 Filariasis

Human filariasis is caused primarily by *Brugia malayi, Onchocerca volvulus* and *Wucheria bancrofti* although 5 other related parasites are pathogenic for humans. Filariasis is endemic in most of Africa, the Far East, and South America. The disease is transmitted to man through the bite of an arthropod vector, most often a mosquito but also *Simulium* spp. (blackflies).

The disease syndrome presented depends upon the infecting parasite and can range from essentially an asymptomatic infection to adenolymphangitis, dermatitis and elephantitis. Infections caused by filarial parasites are often chronic, causing substantial morbidity but little mortality [3]. The adult worms may infest either the lymphatic system, subcutaneous tissues, or body cavities with the exception of *O. volvulus*. Embryos released in the human host mature into microfilariae and enter the bloodstream. It now appears that the majority of symptomatology is due to a vigorous host immune response best illustrated in the case of hypersensitivity characteristic of lymphatic filariasis associated with tropical eosinophilia [4].

The first step in the development of a vaccine against filariasis is to understand the effects that the natural immune response to infection has on the disease course. Following infection, IgG, IgA, IgM and IgE antibody levels to numerous filarial antigens become significantly elevated [5, 6]. In addition to these parasite-specific antibodies, infection also elicits a number of antibodies which crossreact with other filarial species. The relative protective capacities of specific versus cross-reactive antibodies is not known. Similarly, which class of antibody is best able to control the infectious process is also unknown. There is some evidence that IgE has a higher specificity for the infecting parasite than IgG.

The question as to whether humoral antibody is beneficial to the host has not been completely resolved. There appears to be a fine balance between the ability of the host's immune response to control the infection and the induction of an "immune-disease" state. As noted above, a subpopulation of individuals with filariasis will develop hypersensitivity to filarial antigens. In addition, a vigorous antibody response can lead to immune complex formation and attendent pathology [7]. On the positive side, patients with asymptomatic microfilaremia have elevated IgG_4 antibody levels compared to symptomatic patients [8]. Such IgG_4 antibodies were heterogenous as to specificity, recognizing several filarial antigens.

A very encouraging finding is evidence of naturally-acquired immunity among individuals living in an endemic area. A small percentage of adults in such areas are amicrofilaremic without a prior infection [9]. In addition, the prevalence of microfilaremia appears to be age-dependent. Incidence rates increase until age 35 at which time they stabilize or decline slightly.

Recently, several groups have attempted to define "protective filarial antigens" by correlating disease state with antibody levels to a given antigen. Freedman et al. [10] have found that individuals in an endemic area free from infection with *W. bancrofti* have elevated levels of antibody to a 43 kd larval stage antigen. In an independent study, freedom from *W. bancrofti* microfilaremia during infection correlated with increased serum antibody titers to a 25 kd parasite antigen [11].

Infection seems to adversely affect the cell-mediated immune (CMI) response of the host. Infected individuals display a markedly reduced CMI response to both filarial antigens and nonspecific mitogens [12]. Nonresponsiveness is more evident in patients with a high parasite burden and may be due to the generation of a suppressor T-cell population.

Vaccine development is greatly complicated by the fact that each life cycle of the filarial parasite can express numerous antigens. Fortunately, there appears to be considerable crossreactivity at both the species and genus levels [13, 14]. Efforts have therefore centered upon determinating which antigen or antigens would be most effective at inducing a protective immune response be it humoral and/or cellular in nature.

Several studies have shown the ability of human polymorphonuclear leukocytes to kill microfilaria in a complement-dependent fashion in the presence of specific antibodies [15, 16]. However, the critical parasite antigens were not identified. Further evidence to support a key role for antibodies comes from the finding that sera from mice immunized with *B. malayi* microfilarial antigens resulted in a marked decrease in *B. malayi* microfilaremia in recipient mice [17]. Recently, Aggarwal et al. [18] have described a murine monoclonal antibody (MAb) which recognizes a 110 000 dalton antigen on the surface of *B. malayi* microfilaria. This MAb was able to mediate the killing of microfilaria by murine macrophages. When passively transferred to microfilaremic mice, it was able to clear the bloodstream in most (~ 70 %) of the animals. At the present time, it is not known whether the antigen recognized by this MAb is also recognized by the human immune response mounted to natural infection.

Several species of animals can be partially protected against a *B. malayi* or a *B. pahangi* challenge by prior immunization with inactivated larvae [19, 21]. Soluble antigens extracted from *B. malayi* microfilaria can protect mice against challenge. Protection was correlated with an IgG antibody response to several of these antigens [17]. Subsequent studies by this group have shown that serum from animals immunized with inactivated larvae contains antibodies which recognize predominantly 4 microfilarial antigens with a molecular weight of 25, 42, 75 and 150 kilodalton [22]. This antiserum also recognized parasite stages in addition to the microfilaric stage. Nilsen has described the cloning and sequencing of a 60 kd filarial antigen. The gene encoding for this antigen has been expressed in a vaccinia virus vector which was used to immunize jirds. Vaccinated animals showed a markedly reduced level of microfilaremia subsequent to challenge as compared to control animals.

Ideally, a vaccine which prevents infection (anti-larval) is desired. However, an anti-microfilaria vaccine would also be of a considerable advantage since it may not only attenuate disease symptoms but prevent transmission. The finding that antibody to a given parasite stage can also recognize other stages may allow for the development of a single component vaccine able to induce multi-stage immunity.

4.1.3 Schistosomiasis

Human schistosomiasis is caused by *Schistosoma mansoni, S. japonicum* and *S. haematobium* and affects approximately 250 million people living in tropical and sub-tropical areas of the world. Infection occurs by exposure to water containing larvae released by snails, the parasite's intermediate host. After penetration of the skin, the larvae develop into schistosomula which translocate to the liver and lungs. The mature worms then migrate to either the mesenteric veins (*S. mansoni* and *S. japonicum*) or to the vesical plexus veins (*S. haematobium*) where eggs are released. The eggs pass into the intestinal tract and bladder from where they are released via the urine and feces.

Symptoms are usually chronic and charcterized by fever, hepatosplenomegaly, diarrhea and pulmonary dysfunction. However, with *S. japonicum*, acute disease can occur roughly 5-8 weeks post infection. Treatment with chemotherapeutic agents is a long-term process complicated by drug intolerance, toxicity and reinfection.

There is now a consensus that some level of natural immunity, which is age-dependent, can develop in individuals living in an endemic area [23, 24]. Several findings support this conclusion. First, there is an increased level of resistance in persons completing a drug treatment regimen designed to eradicate the parasites [25, 26]. Secondly, superinfection is a rare event in individuals with a primary infection [27]. Finally, there is a marked decrease in the prevalence of infection in individuals living in an endemic area past the age of 25-30 years, which cannot be simply explained by reduced risk of exposure due to behavior modification.

There are several "correlates of immunity" with schistosomiasis. A key factor seems to be the ability of lymphocytes to proliferate in response to exposure to schistosomal antigens [28]. Lymphocytes from patients who were cured by chemotherapy proliferate strongly when exposed to either larval, egg or worm antigens [23]. The degree of proliferation after curing correlates with the level of resistances to subsequent infections. Immune individuals also have increased eosinophil counts compared to non-immune subjects [25].

The immune mechanisms conferring resistances to schistosomiasis are not completely understood. However, immunity is in large part dependent on thymus-specific functions. The best evidence to support this statement is the finding that athymic experimental animals are more susceptible to infection. Surprisingly, lymphoid cells do not appear to be efficient at destroying either mature worms or schistosomula [1]. Antibody-dependent cell-mediated cytotoxicity seems to be the mechanism by which the immune system destroys the invading parasite [1]. Macrophages, and especially eosinophils appear to be the effector cells involved in parasite destruction. Therefore, drug-cured patients with pronounced eosinophilia are highly refractory to reinfection [29].

There is considerable evidence to suggest that antibodies of both the IgE and IgG classes can mediate parasite destruction in cooperation with eosinophils, macrophages and platelets. In Kenyan children, IgG antibody which recognizes an antigen expressed on both schistosomula and eggs can mediate eosinophil-dependent killing of schistosomula [23]. IgG_2 has been shown to be the subclass primarily involved in immunity to schistosomiasis in a rat model [39]. Humans infected with schistosomes mount a vigorous IgE antibody response which is able to trigger cytotoxic killing of schistosomula *in vitro* by various effector cells.

However, certain populations of anti-schistosome antibody appear to interfere with the eradication of the parasite by effector cells. Infection appears to generate a substantial amount of "blocking" antibody, primarily of the IgM class which can inhibit eosinophil-mediated parasite killing. Therefore, IgM antibody from human sera can suppress eosinophil-mediated killing of schistosomula [31]. Furthermore, children in endemic areas who are generally susceptible have elevated levels of such blocking IgM antibodies compared to older resistant individuals.

Adult worms release a substantial amount of soluble antigen which evokes a strong humoral immune response. In chronically infected patients antigen can be found free in serum or in the form of immune complexes [32]. Continued stimulation of the immune system in this way may result in the formation of blocking antibodies and immune complex disease. Furthermore, one may postulate that binding antibody away from the parasite may in itself be a means to avoid a protective immune response.

Based upon the above findings, a vaccine against schistosomiasis should do the following; 1) evoke an antibody response of the proper class and subclass able to mediate antibody-dependent cell-mediated cytotoxicity, and 2) avoid the production of blocking antibodies. This has lead to a concerted effort to identify protective schistosome antigens. A large number of *S. mansoni* antigens have been isolated and characterized [33]. Antibodies to at least 11 such antigens have been shown to provide protection against experimental infections [33]. Many of these antigens have also been successfully used as active immunogens in experimental animal models [33].

The schistosomula of *S. mansoni* appear to express a restricted number of immunogenic surface components [34]. Of these, a 38 kd glycoprotein is of considerable interest since a monoclonal antibody recognizing this antigen is protective [35]. The epitope recognized by this MAb is also expressed by a 115 kd extracellular molecule produced by adult worms. It may therefore induce an antibody response effective against several parasite stages.

A glutathione transferase [GT] from *S. mansoni* has recently been cloned and sequenced [36]. There appears to be considerable antigenic relatedness between GT derived from *S. mansoni* and that derived from *S. japonicum, S. haematobium* and even *S. bovis.* A GT fusion protein was synthesized in *E. coli* and shown to induce good levels of protection in various animal models [36, 2]. The recombinant antigen evoked good levels of IgG antibody which could support eosinophil-dependent killing of parasites. Infected humans possess IgE antibody which recognize cloned GT.

It is foreseeable that one or more of such protective antigens will be evaluated for safety and immunogenicity in humans in the near future. Since schistosomes do not multiply in their human host, even the induction of a partial, non-sterile immune state would be expected to be of considerable benefit.

4.1.4 Cestodiasis (Hydatidosis and Cysticercosis)

Human cestodiasis is caused by infection with the larval stages (metacestodes) of tapeworms belonging to the family of *Taeniidae*. Hydatidosis is caused primarily by *Echinococcus multilocularis* and *E. granulosus*. Humans serve as intermediate hosts and usually become infected by ingesting eggs passed in the feces of the definitive hosts, in this case dogs and foxes. *E. granulosus* can be found worldwide while distribution of *E. multilocularis* is limited to the northern hemisphere. Human cysticercosis is caused by infection with the tapeworm *Taenia solium*. Humans are the definitive host and become infected by ingestion of contaminated pork with pigs serving as the intermediate hosts. *T. solium* is widely distributed, being most prevalent in Asia, Africa and South America.

Disease caused by *E. granulosus* is characterized by the formation of a fluid-filled cyst surrounding the metacestode. Cysts are most frequently located in the liver and lungs although other organs can be affected. *E. multilocularis* initially forms foci of infection in the liver but can also disseminate to other organs. Infection of humans with mature *T. solium* worms is localized to the intestinal tract. Untreated disease can result in a "wasting-disease" syndrome in undernourished individuals. Mild to moderate gastrointestinal symptoms may also be present. A more severe disease syndrome is presented upon metacestode infection of the central nervous system which can result in severe neurological complications.

Repeated infection of intermediate hosts can frequently lead to immunity against subsequent cestode infection. This has stimulated research towards the development of vaccines against cestodes, primarily in the veterinary field. Generally speaking, the control of human cestodiasis may be accomplished by vaccination of humans to prevent infection or by immunization of the animal host to reduce the source of possible infection. The latter approach may prove to be more effective given the low disease incidence in humans and the economic impact of cestode infections in domesticated animals.

Immunization of dogs with secretory antigens of adult tapeworms afforded partial protection against subsequent infection with *E. granulosus* in dogs [37]. Subsequently, Osborn and Heath [38] demonstrated protection against *E. granulosus* in lambs using onchosphere secretory antigens as active immunogens. Neither the nature of the protective antigens nor of the immune response were identified. However, results from studies with *E. multilocularis* suggest that protection is in large part conferred by cell-mediated immunity. Spread of *E. multilocularis* enhanced in thymectomized mice [39]. The growth of *E. multilocularis* metacestodes in mice was reduced in mice immunized with BCG vaccine [40, 41]. In patients with hepatic *Echinococcosis* various activities of T-cells have been shown to be impaired [42].

In attempt to define protective antigens expressed by *E. multilocularis*, Gottstein and coworkers [43] have cloned various *E. multilocularis* genes in *Escherichia coli*. Genes coding for antigens recognized by serum from patients with alveolar echinococcosis were identified by Western blot analysis. A β-galactosidase fusion protein of roughly 130 000 daltons strongly bound antibodies in patient serum but not in control serum or serum infested with *E. granulosus*. This gene was introduced in an attenuated *gal E* mutant strain of *Salmonella typhimurium*. Mice and dogs were vaccinated perorally or subcutaneously with this recombinant strain. In mice, both routes of administration stimulated a serum antibody response and primed lymphocytes to proliferate upon re-exposure to the cloned gene product. A strong humoral antibody response was also noted in dogs. However, only a slight priming of lymphocytes was seen when the vaccine was given subcutaneously. Studies are planned to determine if immunization with this vaccine strain will afford protection against challenge.

Human disease caused by *T. solium* is usually confined to the gastrointestinal tract with symptomatology depending upon the nutritional status of the host. Far less frequent is infection of the central nervous system in the metacestode stage which is accompanied by pronounced morbidity (neurological dysfunction and dementia).

Given the epidemiology of human cysticercosis, it would appear that immunization of the animal intermediate host would be of a greater benefit than to vaccinate humans. Such attempts have recently been reviewed in detail [44].

4.1.5 References

1. Capron, A., Dessaint, J. P., Capron, M., Ouma, J. H. and Butterworth, A. E., *Science* (1987), **238**, 1065-1072.
2. Sasa, M., Human Filariasis. A Global Survey of Epidemiology and Control, Baltimore, MD, University Park Press (1980).
3. Nelson, G. S., *N. Engl. J. Med.* (1979), **300**, 1136-1140.
4. Otteson, E. A., Nera, F. A., Paranjape, R. S., Tripathy, S. P., Thisurengadam, K. V. and Beaven, M. A., *Lancet* (1979), **i**, 1158-1161.
5. Akiyama, T., Ushijima, N., Anan, S., Nonoka, S., Yoshida, H. and Flores, G. E. Z., *J. Dermatol.* (1981), **8**, 43-46.
6. Greene, B. M., Gbakima, A. A., Albiez, E. J. and Taylor, H. R., *Rev. Infect. Dis.* (1985), **7**, 789-795.
7. Steward, M. W., Sisley, B., Mackenzie, C. D. and El-Sheik, H. E., *Clin. Exp. Immunol.* (1982), **48**, 17-24.
8. Hussain, R., Grögl, M. and Ottesen, E. A., *J. Immunol.* (1987), **139**, 2794-2798.
9. World Health Organization, *WHO Document TDR/FIL/SWG (13)* **87.3**, *Geneva, Switzerland* (1987).
10. Freedman, D. O., Nutman, T. B. and Ottesen, E. A., *J. Clin. Invest.* (1989), **83**, 14-22.
11. Kazura, J. W., Cicirello, H. and Forsyth, K. P., *J. Clin. Invest.* (1986), **77**, 1985-1992.
12. Piessens, W. F., Partono, F., Hoffman, S. L., Ratiwayanto, S., Piessens, P. W., Palmieri, J. R., Koiman, I., Dennis, D. T. and Carney, W. P., *N. Engl. J. Med.* (1982), **307**, 144-148.
13. Lal, R. B. and Ottesen, E. A., *J. Immunol.* (1988), **140**, 2032-2038.
14. Selkirk, M. E., Denham, D. A., Partono, F., Sutanto, I. and Maizels, R. M., *Parasitology* (1986), **91**, S15-S38.
15. Greene, B. M., Taylor, H. R. and Aikawa, M., *J. Immunol.* (1981), **127**, 1611-1616.
16. Simonsen, P. E., *Trans. R. Soc. Trop. Med. Hyg.* (1983), **77**, 289-296.
17. Kazura, J. W. and Davis, R. S., *J. Immunol.* (1982), **128**, 1792-1796.
18. Aggarwal, A., Cuna, W., Haque, A., Dissous, C. and Capron, A., *Immunol.* (1985), **54**, 655-663.
19. Hayashi, Y., Noda, K., Shirasaka, A., Nogami, S. and Nakamura, M., *Jpn. J. Exp. Med.* (1984), **54**, 177-181.
20. Oothuman, P., Denham, D. A., McGreevy, P. B., Nelson, G. S. and Rogers, R., *Parasite Immunol.* (1979), **1**, 209-215.
21. Wong, M. M., Fredericks, H. J. and Ramachandran, C. P., *Bull. WHO* (1969), **40**, 493-501.
22. Kazura, J. W., Cicerello, H. and McCall, J. W., *J. Immunol.* (1986), **136**, 1422-1426.
23. Butterworth, A. E. and Hagan, P., *Parasitology Today* (1987), **3**, 11-16.

24. Capron, A., Dessaint, J. P., Capron, M., Ouma, J. H. and Butterworth, A. E., *Science* (1987), **238**, 1065-1072.
25. Hagan, P., Wilkins, H. A., Blumenthal, U. J., Hayes, R. J. and Greenwood, B. M., *Parasite Immunol.* (1985), **7**, 625-632.
26. von Lichtenberg, F., *Am. J. Trop. Med. Hyg.* (1985), **34**, 78-85.
27. Wilkins, H. A., Goll, P. H., Marshall de C., T. F. and Moore, P. J., *Trans. R. Soc. Trop. Med. Hyg.* (1984), **78**, 227-232.
28. Todd, C. W., Goodgame, R. W. and Colley, D. G., *J. Immunol.* (1979), **122**, 1440-1446.
29. Sturrock, R. F., Kimani, R., Cottrell, B. J., Butterworth, A. E., Seitz, H. M., Siongok, T. K. and Houba, V., *Trans. R. Soc. Trop. Med. Hyg.* (1983), **77**, 363-371.
30. Capron, M., Capron, A., Torpier, G., Bazin, H., Bout, D. and Joseph, M., *Europ. J. Immunol.* (1978), **8**, 127-133.
31. Khalife, J., Capron, M., Capron, A., Grzych, J.-M., Butterworth, A. E., Dunne, D. W. and Ouma, J. H., *J. Exp. Med.* (1986), **164**, 1626-1640.
32. Steens, W. J., Feldmeir, H., Bridts, C. H. and Daffalla, A. A., *Clin. Exp. Immunol.* (1983), **52**, 142-152.
33. Simpson, A. J. G. and Cioli, D., *Parasitology Today* (1987), **3**, 26-28.
34. Dissous, C., Dissous, C. and Capron, A., *Mol. Biochem. Parasitol.* (1981), **3**, 215-225.
35. Dissous, C., Grzych, M. and Capron, A., *J. Immunol.* (1982), **129**, 2232-2234.
36. Balloul, J. M., Sondermeyer, P., Dreyer, D., Capron, M., Grzych, J. M., Pierce, R. J., Carvallo, D., Lecocq, J. P. and Capron, A., *Nature* (1987), **326**, 149-153.
37. Herd, R. P., Chappel, R. J. and Biddell, D., *Int. J. Parasitol.* (1975), **5**, 395-399.
38. Osborn, J. J. and Heath, D. D., *Res. Vet. Sci.* (1982), **33**, 132-133.
39. Baron, R. W. and Tanner, C. E., *Int. J. Parasitol.* (1976), **6**, 37-42.
40. Rau, M. E. and Tanner, C. E., *Nature* (1975), **256**, 318-319.
41. Reubin, J. M. and Tanner, C. E., *Parasite Immunol.* (1983), **5**, 61-66.
42. Vuitton, D., Lassegue, A., Miguet, J. P., Herve, P., Barale, T., Seilles, E. and Capron, A., *Parasite Immunol.* (1984), **6**, 329-340.
43. Gottstein, B., Müller, N., Cryz, S. J., Jr., Vogel, M., Tanner, T. and Seebeck, T., *Parasite Immunol.* (1989), in press.
44. Rickard, M. D. and Williams, J. F. *Adv. Parasitol.* (1982), **21**, 229-296.

4.2 Malaria Vaccine

L. H. Perrin

Malaria remains a major health problem in many tropical and subtropical countries and affects hundreds of million of people each year. A major effort was made to control malaria from 1950-1970 with insecticides and antimalarial drugs. The initial remarkable results have been difficult to maintain. The emergence of drug-resistant parasite strains and of insecticide-resistant mosquito vectors are major obstacles in the effort to control malaria. Since the early 1970s new approaches have been explored such as vector control through biological agents and control of malaria infection through vaccines.

The development of malaria vaccine has received considerable impetus: first, because immunization of animals with whole parasites can induce a degree of protection equal or superior to that induced following natural infection [1-3]; second, because *in vitro* culture systems have been developed for the blood and hepatic stages of the malarial parasite *Plasmodium falciparum* [4, 5]; and third, because monoclonal antibody and recombinant DNA techniques have been used to identify and produce the parasite polypeptides possibly involved in the development of protective immunity.

4.2.1 Strategy for Malaria Vaccine Development

More than 100 species of malarial plasmodia are known, but only four infect humans: *Plasmodium falciparum*, which is responsible for the majority of human deaths, *P. vivax, P. malariae* and *P. ovale*.

The life cycle of the plasmodia is complex (Fig. 4-1). The female anopheline mosquitoes inoculate *sporozoites* into the blood of the vertebrate host. Within minutes the sporozoites invade the liver parenchymal cells (hepatocytes) where they divide asexually and develop into *merozoites* which rupture the hepatocytes and reenter the blood. In the subsequent *erythrocytic cycle,* the merozoites invade the red blood cells and mature into *schizonts* within 48-72 h depending on the species. The mature schizonts release merozoites which invade new erythrocytes. The erythrocytic cycle is responsible for the clinical manifestations of malaria. Some merozoites differentiate into sexual stages called *gametocytes* which are ingested by the mosquito. Fertilization of the gametes occurs solely in the midgut of the mosquito. The resulting zygotes develop into *ookinetes* and then into *oocysts.* Sporozoites are released from mature oocysts and migrate to the mosquito salivary glands. The cycle is then repeated.

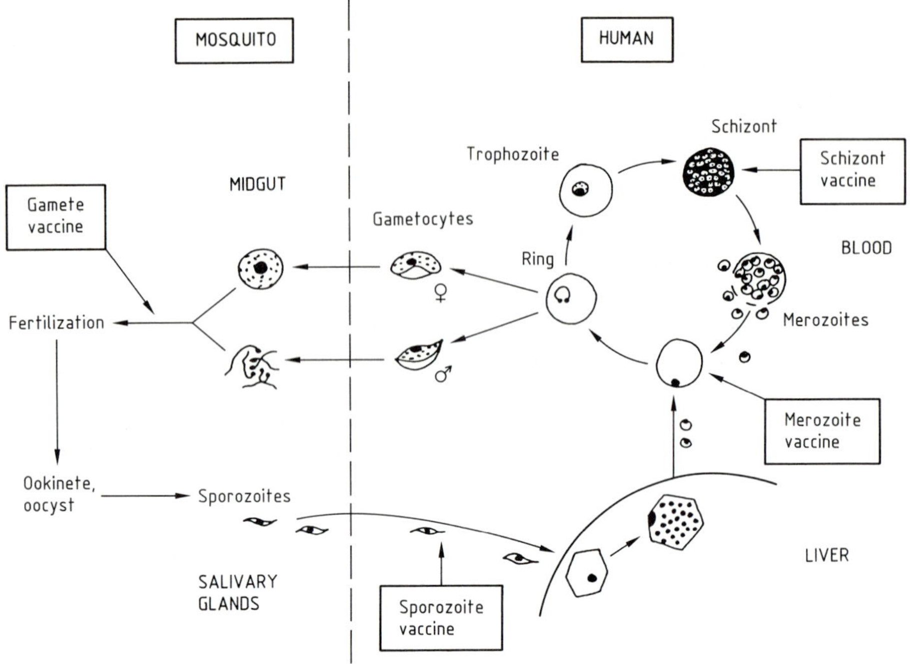

Fig. 4-1 *Plasmodium falciparum* life cycle showing targets for vaccine development.

This complex life cycle involves continuous morphologic, enzymatic, and antigenic changes which are linked to the parasite's environmental adaptation to the host. The invasive stages of the parasite (sporozoites, merozoites, gametes) have unique, stage-specific surface determinants. Furthermore, immunologic crossreactivity exists between plasmodia species and between the developmental stages of a given species. However, immunization experiments in animal models have demonstrated that the antigenic determinants involved in protective responses are species- and stage-specific. Three types of malaria vaccine can therefore be devised based on:

1) sporozoites,
2) asexual stages (merozoites, schizonts) and
3) sexual stages (gametes).

In addition, recent data indicate that stage-specific parasitic antigens are expressed on liver cells containing merozoites [8] and may also be candidates for vaccine development. A favored approach is the development of a multivalent vaccine containing components of several malaria stages. The selection of defined parasite components versus whole parasites (sporozoites, merozoites, gametes) for vaccine development is indicated by the following reasons:

1) Large-scale production and purification of whole parasites is not feasible.
2) Parasites cannot be obtained free of host components (e. g., mosquito salivary glands, erythrocyte membranes) which may induce adverse autoimmune reactions.
3) Most of the parasite components are irrelevant to the induction of a protective response and their inclusion may impair truly protective responses or induce immunopathologic lesions in the host.

The current strategy for the development of malaria vaccine is as follows:

1) Identification and selection of malaria antigens that are the target of protective immune responses.
2) Functional, biochemical, and immunological characterization of these antigens, including identification of B and T cell epitopes.
3) Cloning of the genes coding for protective antigens, determination of DNA and amino acid sequences - what is the level of antigenic diversity?
4) Production of candidate protective antigens or epitopes by genetic engineering or chemical synthesis.
5) Evaluation of candidate protective antigens in terms of production of antigens, safety tests, adjuvants, carriers, etc.
6) Immunization trials in monkeys and human volunteers.

4.2.2 Sporozoite Vaccines

Following invasion of the hepatocytes, the sporozoites develop into thousands of merozoites, each of which may invade an erythrocyte. Obviously a vaccine which neutralizes sporozoites before their entry into liver cells or within liver cells would optimally prevent malaria infection. Vaccination with attenuated, irradiated sporozoites in rodents, monkeys, and humans induced complete protection against malaria [7, 8]. The induced immunity is species- and stage-specific but not strain-specific. It is at least partially mediated by antibodies as is shown by protection against sporozoite challenge afforded by the passive transfer of antisporozoite monoclonal antibody [13] and by neutralization of sporozoite infectivity following incubation with the serum of protected animals. Deposition of specific antibodies on the sporozoite surface results in the formation of a tail-like precipitate; this is called the circumsporozoite (CS) reaction. Indirect evidence suggests that antisporozoite antibodies may play a role in human malaria [9, 10].

The control of sporozoite-induced infection also involves T cell-dependent mechanisms. In animal models, effector T cells can mediate antisporozoite immunity via antibody-independent mechanisms; for example, immunization with irradiated sporozoites can protect B cell-deficient mice against subsequent challenge infection with viable sporozoites [11]. Activation of malaria-specific T cells by malaria antigens induces the secretion of lymphokines which may act directly on the malaria parasite or indirectly by activating host effector systems [12].

The CS protein has been identified in several plasmodia species. Passive transfer of monoclonal antibodies directed against the CS protein protects mice from sporozoite challenge infection [13]. Indirect evidence suggests that CS protein is involved in the binding and penetration of sporozoites into liver cells. Similarly, fragments of monoclonal antibodies against CS prevent the attachment of sporozoites to hepatocytes *in vitro* [14].

The gene coding for the CS protein has been cloned in several plasmodial species [15, 16]. The protein contains a central block of tandemly repeated amino acids which vary in number and sequence among the different malaria species [17, 18]. For example, in *P. falciparum* the central area consists of 37 copies of the tetrapeptide asparagine-alanine-asparagine-proline (NANP) and four copies of the tetrapeptide asparagine-valine-aspartic acid-proline (NVDP). The regions flanking the repeats are more highly conserved between species than the repeats. Within a species, limited variations also occur outside the repeats [19].

The repeats cover the surface of mature sporozoites; for *P. falciparum* ca. 10^8 molecules of NANP are expressed on the membrane of mature sporozoites. The NANP repeats are the target of protective monoclonal antibodies passively transferred *in vivo*. The antibody response against sporozoites in humans is also mainly directed against the NANP repeats [20, 21]

In view of these findings, and because the NANP repeats are present on all the isolates of *P. falciparum* tested, two malaria vaccines based on NANP repeats have been prepared and tested on human volunteers. The first, produced by DNA recombinant technology, consisted of 32 repeats of NANP and NVDP fused to a 32 amino acid tail. The second was composed of three NANP repeats (NANP 3) conjugated to tetanus toxoid. Both formulations use aluminium hydroxide as adjuvant [22, 23]. The vaccines were safe and did not induce adverse reactions. Volunteers with high antisporozoite antibody titers were challenged with sporozoites and some were protected or presented a delay in appearance of parasitemia. Protection was shown in individuals with the highest antibody titers.

An antisporozoite vaccine must induce high antibody titers for a prolonged period and ideally a boostering effect should occur following exposure to sporozoites. Higher antibody responses can be obtained by changing the formulation and concentration of the immunogens and by using other adjuvants or live-attenuated vectors (vaccinia virus, *Salmonella*) that carry and express the gene coding for the CS protein. Optimal antibody formation is dependent on the collaboration of T helper cells and B cells. In the two sporozoite vaccines tested, T cell help was provided by foreign protein (tetanus toxoid) but was unable to boost the anti NANP antibody response following exposure to sporozoites. More efficient sporozoite vaccines should contain T cell epitopes derived from sporozoites and ideally from the CS protein; in this context, proper help is provided by sporozoite-specific, primed T cells and can lead to optimal anti NANP antibody production by B cells. In a mouse model the response to some of the T cell epitopes of the CS protein is restricted by antigens of the major histo-compatibility complex (MHC class II) [24-27]. In human populations, only three immunodominant epitopes are located in polymorphic regions of the CS protein outside the repetitive area. Since T cells have exquisitely specific reactivity, it follows that the polymorphism of T cell determinants may be responsible for a lack of proper help following exposure to sporozoites with T cell areas on CS that are different from those present on sporozoites responsible for previous infections in the same individual.

Therefore, it seems that more efficient vaccines should be based on either native malaria polypeptide(s) or cocktails of synthetic polypeptides containing multiple B and T cell epitopes. These epitopes should be selected in relation to constant and variant parasite components and in relation to epitope binding and recognition by components of the major histocompatibility complex of the human host.

4.2.3 Asexual Blood Stage Vaccine

The multiplication of asexual blood stages (merozoites and schizonts) is responsible for the morbidity and mortality associated with malaria. The level of parasitemia usually correlates with the severity of malaria infection. Immunity to malaria is mostly acquired but natural immunity also plays a role. Several single-gene disorders affecting erythrocytes, (e. g., sickle cell anemia, the thalassemias, and glucose phosphate deficiency) reduce the severity of malaria infection. Another genetic characteristic, the lack of the Duffy blood group antigens, is associated with complete resistance to *P. vivax* infection [28]; the Duffy blood group antigen or a closely associated antigen may be the receptor for *P. vivax* merozoites at the surface of erythrocytes.

The development of acquired resistance to malaria depends on the frequency and duration of the exposure to the parasite [29]. In endemic areas, babies born to immune mothers are resistant to malaria during the first three months of life due to the presence of maternal antibodies transferred during gestation. Later they suffer from severe, recurrent attacks, most deaths due to malaria occur in young children. From adolescence to adulthood there is a decrease in the severity and frequency of malaria attacks but sterile immunity is probably never achieved. In this context two types of vaccine based on asexual blood stages can be envisaged; (1) a vaccine which is more efficient than nature and leads to sterile immunity (i. e., infection no longer detectable) or (2) a vaccine capable of attenuating the parasite load by transforming the immune system of a non-immune individual into that of an adult living in an endemic area.

The immune response to blood stages is complex and is directed against several antigens. Both antibody-mediated responses and cell-mediated, antibody-independent responses control asexual blood-stage infection. In humans, passive transfer of immunoglobulins purified from the sera of immune adults abort malaria infection in non-immune infected children [30]. The antibodies may react with the surface of the merozoites and provoke their lysis upon addition of complement, or enhance their phagocytosis by mononuclear cells, or simply inhibit the binding of merozoites to erythrocytes. Other targets for antibodies are antigens on the surface of erythrocytes containing schizonts; binding of antibodies to schizonts may also lead to their destruction by phagocytosis [31] or induce the endothelial release of schizonts which may be later destroyed in the spleen [32]. Immunity to asexual blood stages also operates through a variety of antibody-independent mechanisms: T cell-dependent release of lymphokines, induction of oxidizing radicals leading to intracellular death of the malaria parasites, and activation of mononuclear cells in the spleen.

Immunization with merozoites and/or schizonts in a variety of plasmodia-host systems resulted in partial to almost complete protection [33]. Subsequent investigations were aimed at the characterization of components capable of inducing immunity. Several hundreds of asexual blood stage components can raise an immune response but only very few of the evoked responses are helpful to the host. Characteristics of some of the candidate antigens for asexual bloodstage vaccines are discussed in sections 4.2.3.1-4.2.3.4.

4.2.3.1 Merozoite Surface Antigens

A protein with a molecular mass of 190-200 kDa has been identified at the surface of *P. falciparum* schizonts and merozoites [34, 35]. During maturation of schizonts this polypeptide is processed into several components, one of them (M_r 83 000) Being the main surface component of the merozoites [35]. An important feature of the 190-200 kDa protein is its genetic polymorphism [35-39]. The gene coding for the protein can be divided into blocks ranging in homology among different *P. falciparum* isolates from 10-87 % at the amino acid level. A relatively short region of variable tripeptide repeats is found close to the N terminus. The blocks encoding for the N and C terminal sequences are highly conserved.

Immunization with the 190-200 kDa protein derived from *P. falciparum* in monkeys [40-42] and with an analogous protein from *P. voelii* [43] can induce at least partial protection. Immunization with synthetic polypeptides corresponding to defined parts of the molecule (for example, the N terminus and amino acids 277-278) also confer partial protection in monkeys [44, 45].

An antigen with a molecular mass of 51 kDa is also expressed at the surface of *P. falciparum* merozoites and is the target of inhibitory monoclonal antibodies. It contains variant and constant epitopes for various *P. falciparum* isolates.

There is considerable antigenic diversity among *P. vivax* isolates as regards the components exposed at the surface of merozoites.

4.2.3.2 Rhoptry Antigens

Rhoptries are apical organelles of the merozoites which release their contents onto the erythrocyte membrane during invasion. A monoclonal antibody directed against a rhoptry protein of a rodent malaria, *P. yoelii*, reduced the virulence of the infection and a monoclonal antibody directed against 82 and 41 kDa components of *P. falciparum* inhibited the growth of *P. falciparum in vitro* [46-48]. The 82 kDa component is processed into 82 and 65 kDa components [49].

The 82 kDa polypeptide is membrane-bound through a glycosyl-phosphatide-inositol anchor; hydrolysis of its anchor activates the proteolytic activity of the 76 kDa polypeptide and may play a role in the invasion of erythrocytes by merozoites [50]. The 41 kDa polypeptide displays aldolase activity [51]. Interestingly, both the 76 kDa and the 41 kDa components can induce at least partial protection against *P. falciparum* infection in monkeys [52, 53]. The gene coding for the 41 kDa protein has been cloned and presents two interesting characteristics in terms of vaccine development; absence of variable amino acid repeats and almost complete conservation of the amino acid sequences among isolates from *P. falciparum* [51].

Another rhoptry antigen of *P. falciparum* with a molecular mass of 225 kDa has been identified in the peduncle of the rhoptries. It is synthesized as a 240 kDa polypeptide which is processed into a 225 kDa protein during schizogony and is quantitatively recovered in the culture supernatant following merozoite invasion [54].

A third set of rhoptry-associated proteins is the 105-130-140 kDa complex composed of three coprecipitating but unrelated proteins [55]. The 225 kDa proteins and the 105-130-140 kDa complex have not been evaluated in immunization trials.

4.2.3.3 Antigens Associated with the Membrane of Infected Erythrocytes

The ring-infected erythrocyte surface antigen (RESA) is a *P. falciparum* antigen with a molecular mass of 155 kDa. It is synthesized in trophozoites, accumulates in the merozoite, and, following invasion, becomes associated with the membrane of erythrocytes containing ring forms of the parasite [56, 57], but is not directly accessible on the external erythrocyte surface. Anti-RESA antibodies inhibit the multiplication of asexual blood stages *in vitro* and may interfere with the invasion process [58]. The gene coding for RESA has been cloned and sequenced [59]. It contains two blocks of repetitive amino acid sequences which are the immunodominant regions of the molecule in terms of antibody response. Antibodies directed against the RESA repeats crossreact with at least six other asexual blood stage components. Aotus monkeys have been immunized with fusion proteins corresponding to various areas of the RESA and with synthetic polypeptides corresponding to the repetitive sequences [60]. Partial protection was observed in some groups of animals; work is in progress to optimize the efficacy of immunization based on RESA-derived molecules.

Erythrocytes containing mature asexual blood stages of *P. falciparum* attach to endothelial cells lining the venules of deep tissues. This cytoadherence of mature parasites prevents their passage through the spleen and thus their exposure to localized destructive mechanisms. Electron-dense protuberances (knobs) on the plasma membranes of infected erythrocytes are implicated in cytoadherence [61]. The genes coding for two knob components (knob-associated histidine-rich protein M_r 85-105 kDa) and mature parasite-infected erythrocyte surface antigen M_r 240-300 kDa) have been cloned [62, 63]. The two proteins differ antigenically among isolates and contain repeated amino acid sequences. Cytoadherence can be inhibited by antisera in a strain-specific manner [64]. However, an antigenically invariant epitope has also been identified on the surface of infected erythrocyte isolates and may be an important antigen for vaccine development [65].

4.2.3.4 Other Proteins and Synthetic Peptides

A number of other antigens are also candidates for vaccine development. *P. falciparum* requires exogenous iron in the form of ferrotransferrin. A malaria transferrin receptor at the surface of infected erythrocytes transports bound ferrotransferrin to the parasite and may be used as a target for the vaccine [66]. Glycophorins exposed at the erythrocyte surface may act as ligands for *P. falciparum* merozoites and *P. falciparum* proteins have been identified which either bind to glycophorins or to human erythrocytes [67, 68]. A prominent antigen of *P. falciparum* with an apparent molecular mass of 126-140 kDa is associated with merozoite release. The gene coding for this protein has been cloned and contains at least two stretches of amino acid repeats, one being composed of polyserine repeats [69]. Monkeys immunized with this protein are protected from a lethal challenge infection [40].

Several immunization trials have been conducted in monkeys using synthetic peptides derived from asexual blood stages of *P. falciparum* coupled to carrier proteins [43, 44, 60]. A partial protective response was observed with peptides corresponding to various areas of the 190-200 kDa protein, to RESA, and to fragments of parasite components identified by their molecular mass of 55 and 35 kDa [44]. Recently synthetic hybrid polymer-proteins containing several peptides corresponding to epitopes of the 195-200 kDa, RESA, 55 kDa, 35 kDa, and CS proteins have been used for immunization human volunteers [69]. The vaccine was well tolerated and no adverse effects were observed. All the immunized and control volunteers had latent parasitemia but the majority of the immunized volunteers were able to control their parasitemia in the absence of drug therapy. The immune response was low in terms of specific antibody production, and cell mediated responses as measured by proliferation assays were undetectable.

4.2.4 Sexual Stages - Transmission Blocking Immunity

The transmission of malaria from the vertebrate host to the mosquito vector is effected by sexual parasite stages - the gametocytes - which develop from merozoites. Within the vertebrate host the gametocytes are surrounded by the erythrocyte membrane; following ingestion by the mosquito vector, the female gametes are fertilized by the male gametes in the midgut of the mosquito to produce zygotes which develop into ookinetes. The ookinetes penetrate the midgut wall where they remain to form oocysts in which the sporozoites develop.

In the vertebrate host, the sexual stages do not produce illness, and their intracellular localization prevents direct attack by host effector mechanisms. Within the midgut of the mosquito the extracellular gametes are exposed to antigamete and/or antizygote antibodies from the vertebrate host that are ingested with the mosquito's blood meal. The antibodies partially or completely prevent the development of sexual stages and subsequent production of sporozoites. Transmission of the parasites is therefore blocked. This phenomenon is termed *transmission blocking immunity.*

The development of vaccines based on sexual blood stages could have an important impact on the epidemiology of malaria in endemic areas by reducing the level of malaria transmission. Ideally, transmission blocking vaccines have to be used in combination with vaccines based on sporozoite and/or asexual blood stages (see sections 4.2.2 and 4.2.3).

Transmission blocking immunity has been induced by immunization with extracellular gametes in several animals [70-73]. The induced antigamete response is long lasting and in some cases is boostered by malaria infection, probably due to the gametocyte antigens in the circulation of the vertebrate host [73, 74]. There is also evidence that in *P. vivax* malaria in humans the antigamete response is boostered during natural infection [75]. Addition of sera of previously infected individuals to gametes can prevent fertilization and development of oocysts in mosquitos.

Specific targets for antigamete immunity have been identified using monoclonal antibodies in species including the human parasites *P. falciparum* and *P. vivax* [76, 77]. The antibodies act against the gametes by preventing fertilization and against the zygotes and ookinetes by preventing further development. In *P. falciparum* the target antigens for inhibition of fertilization are polypeptides with a molecular mass of 230 kDa and 45-48 kDa [76, 77]. Some of the epitopes on the 45-48 kDa antigen have been defined and are the targets of inhibitory monoclonal antibodies [78]. New antigens are expressed at the surface of the zygote and ookinete and one of them (M_r = 25 kDa) is a probable target of inhibitory monoclonal antibodies [76].

4.2.5 References

1. Nussenzweig, R. S., Vanderberg, H., Most, H. and Orton, C., *Nature* (1967), **216**, 160-162.
2. Siddiqui, W. A., *Science* (1977), **197**, 388-389.
3. Mitchell, G. H., Richards, W. H. G., Butcher, G. A. and Cohen, S., *Lancet* (1977), **i**, 1335-1358.
4. Trager, W. and Jensen, J. B., *Science* (1976), **193**, 673-675.
5. Mazier, D., Beaudoin, R. L., Mellouk, S., Druilhe, P., et al., *Science* (1985), **227**, 440-442.
6. Guerin-Marchand, C., Druilhe, P., Galey, B., Londono, A., et al., *Nature* (1987), **329**, 164-167.
7. Cochrane, A. H., *In:* Kreier, J. P. (ed.), Malaria Immunology and Immunization, **vol. 3, chap. 4**, Academic-Press, New York (1980).
8. Clyde, D. F., *Am. J. Trop. Med. Hyg.* (1975), **24**, 397-401.
9. Nardin, E. H., Nussenzweig, R. S., McGregor, I. A. and Bryan, J. H., *Science* (1979), **206**, 597-599.
10. del Giudice, G., Engers, H. D., Tougne, C., Biro, S. S., et al., *Am. J. Trop. Med. Hyg.* (1987), **36**, 203-212.
11. Chen, D. H., Tigelaar, R. E. and Weinbaum, P. I. , *J. Immunol.* (1977), **118**, 1322-1327.
12. Ferreira, A., Schofield, L., Enea, V., Schellekins, H., et al., *Science* (1986), **232**, 881-884.
13. Potocnjak, P., Yoshida, N., Nussenzweig, R. S. and Nussenzweig, V., *J. Exp. Med.* (1980), **151**, 1504-1513.
14. Mazier, D., Mellouk, S., Beaudoin, R. L., Texier, B., et al., *Science* (1986), **231**, 156-159.
15. Dame, J. B., Williams, J. L., McCutchan, T. F., Weber, J. L., et al., *Science* (1984), **225**, 593-599.
16. Enea, V., Ellis, J., Zavala, F., Arnot, D. E., et al. *Science* (1984), **225**, 628-630.
17. Kemp, D. J., Coppel, R. L. and Anders, R. F., *Ann. Rev. Microbiol.* (1987), **41**, 181-208.
18. de la Cruz, V. F., Lal, A. A. and McCutchan, T. F., *J. Biol. Chem.* (1987), **262**, 11935-11941.
19. Lockyer, M. J. and Schwarz, R. T., *Mol. Biochem. Parasitol* (1987), **22**, 101-107.
20. del Guidice, G., Verdini, A. S., Pinori, M., Verhave, J. P., et al., *J. Clin. Microbiol.* (1987), **25**, 91-96.
21. Hoffman, S. L., Wistar, R., Jr., Ballou, W. R., Hollingdale, M. R., et al., *New-Engl. J. Med.* (1986), **315**, 601-603.
22. Herrington, D. A., Clyde, D. F., Losonsky, G., Cortesia, M.et al., *Nature* (1987), **328**, 257-259.
23. Ballou, W. R., Hoffman, S. L., Sherwood, J. A., Hollingdale, M. R., et al., *Lancet* (1987), **i**, 1277-1279.
24. del Guidice, G., Cooper, J. A., Merino, J., Verdini, A. S., et al., *J. Immunol.* (1986), **137**, 2952-2955.
25. Good, M. F., Berzofsky, J. A., Maloy, W. L., Hayashi, Y., et al., *J. Exp. Med.* (1986), **164**, 655-660.
26. Togna, A. R., del Duidice, G., Verdini, A. S., Bonetti, F., et al., *J. Immunol. (1986),* **137**, 2956-2960.
27. Good, M. F., Pombo, D., Quakyi, I. A., Riley E. M., et al., *Proc. Natl. Acad. Sci. U.S.A.* (1988), **85**, 1199-1203.

28. Miller, L. H., Mason, S. J., Clyde, D. F. and McGinis, M. H., *Trans. Roy. Soc. Trop. Med. Hyg.* (1976), **295**, 302-304.
29. Miller, M. J., *Trans. Roy. Soc. Trop. Med. Hyg.* (1958), **52**, 152-158.
30. Cohen, S., McGregor, I. A. and Carrington, S. C., *Nature* (1961), **192**, 733-735.
31. Celada, A., Cruchau, A. and Perrin, L. H., *Clin. Exp. Immunol.* (1982), **47**, 635-641.
32. David, P. H., *Proc. Natl. Acad. Sci. U.S.A.* (1983), **80**, 5075-5081.
33. Miller, L. H., Howard, R. J., Carter, R., Good, M. F., et al., *Science* (1986), **234**, 1349-1356.
34. Perrin, L. H., Ramirez, E., Er-Hsiang, L. and Lambert, P.-H., *Clin. Exp. Immunol.* (1980), **41**, 91-106.
35. Holder, A. A. and Freeman, R. R., *J. Exp. Med.* (1982), **156**, 1528-1538.
36. McBride, J. S., Walliker, D. and Morgan, G., *Science* (1982), **217**, 254-256.
37. Holder, A. A., Lockyer, M. J., Odink, K. G., Sandhu, J. S., et al., *Nature* (1985), **317**, 270-273.
38. Oding, K. G., Lockyer, M. J., Nicholls, S. C., Hillman, Y., et al., *FEBS Lett.* (1984), **173**, 108-112.
39. Mackay, M., Goman, M., Bone, N., Hyde, J. E., et al., *EMBO J.* (1985), **4**, 3823-3829.
40. Perrin, L. H., Merkli, B, Loche, M., Chizzolini, C., et al., *J. Exp. Med.* (1984), **160**, 441-447.
41. Hall, R., Hyde, J. E., Goman, M., Simmons, D. L., et al., *Nature* (1984), **311**, 379-382.
42. Siddiqui, W. A., Tam, L. Q., Kramer, K. J., Hui, G. S. N., et al., *Proc. Natl. Acad. Sci. U.S.A.* (1987), **84**, 3014-3018.
43. Holder, A. A. and Freeman, R. R., *Nature* (1981), **294**, 361-363.
44. Patarroyo, M. E., Romero, P., Torres, M. L., Clavijo, P., et al., *Nature* (1985), **328** , 629-631.
45. Cheung, A., Leban, J., Shaw, A. R., Merkli, B., et al., *Proc. Natl. Acad. Sci. U.S.A.* (1986), **83**, 8323-8332.
46. Perrin, L. H. and Dayal, R., *Immunol. Rev.* (1982), **61**, 245-268.
47. Freeman, R. R., Trejosiewicz, A. J. and Cross, G. A., *Nature* (1980), **284**, 366-369.
48. Perrin, L. H., Ramirez, E., Lambert, P.-H. and Miescher, P. A., *Nature* (1981), **289**, 301-303.
49. Braun-Breton, C., Jendoubi, M., Brunet, E., Perrin, L., et al., *Mol. Bioch. Parasitol.* (1986), **20**, 33-38.
50. Braun-Breton, C., Rosenberg, T. L. and Pereira Da Silva, L., *Nature* (1988), **332**, 457-459.
51. Certa, U., Ghersa, P., Dobeli, H., Matile, H., et al., *Science* (1988), **240**, 1036-1038.
52. Dubois, P., Dedet, J. P., Fandeur, T., Roussilhon, C., et al., *Proc. Natl. Acad. Sci. U.S.A.* (1984), **81**, 229-335.
53. Perrin, L. H., Merkli, B., Gabra, M. S., Stocker, J., et al., *J. Clin. Invest.* (1985), **75**, 1718-1725.
54. Dubremetz, J. F., Delplace, P., Fortier, B., Tronchin, G., et al., *Mol. Biochem. Parasitol.* (1988), **27**, 135-142.
55. Coppel, R. L., Culvenor, J. G., Bianco, A. E., Crewther, P. E., et al., *Mol. Biochem. Parasitol.* (1987), **25**, 73-81.
56. Perlamnn, H., Berzins, K., Wahlgren, M., Carlsson, J., et al., *J. Exp. Med.* (1984), **159**, 1686-1693.
57. Brown, G. V., Culvenor, I. G., Crewther, P. E., Bianco, A. E., et al., *J. Exp. Med.* (1985), **162**, 774-779.
58. Wahlin, B., Wahlgren, M., Perlamnn, H. Berzins, H., et al., *Proc. Natl. Acad. Sci. U.S.A.* (1984), **81**, 7912-7916.
59. Favarolo, J. M., Coppel, R. L., Corcoran, L. M., Foote, S. J., et al., *Nucl. Acid. Res.* (1986), **14**, 8265-8277.
60. Collins, W. E., Anders, R. F., Pappaioanou, M., Campbell, G. H., et al., *Nature* (1986), **323**, 259-262.
61. Luse, S. A. and Miller, L. H., *Am. J. Trop. Med. Hyg.* (1971), **20**, 655-670.
62. Triglia, T., Stahl, H. D., Crewther, P. E., Scanlon, D., et al., *EMBO J.* (1987), **6**, 1413-1419.
63. Koenen, M., Scherf, A., Mercereau, O., Langsley, G., et al., *Nature* (1984), **311**, 382-385.
64. Udeinya, I. J., Miller, L. H. McGregor, I. A., Jensen, J. B., et al., *Nature* (1983), **231**, 429-431.
65. Marsh, K. and Howard, R. J., *Science* (1986), **231**, 150-153.
66. Pollack, S. and Fleming, J., *Brit. J. Haematol.* (1984), **58**, 289-294.
67. Perkins, M. E., *J. Exp. Med.* (1984), **160**, 788-797.
68. Camus, D. and Hadley, T. J., *Science* (1985), **230**, 553-557.

69. Delplace, P., Fortier, B., Tronchin, G., Dubremetz, J. F., et al., *Mol. Biochem. Parasitol.* (1987), **23**, 193-202.
70. Patarroyo, M. E., Amador, R., Lvijo, P., Moreno, A., et al., *Nature* (1988), **332**, 158-161.
71. Gwadz, R. W., *Science* (1976), **193**, 1150-1153.
72. Mendis, K. N. and Targett, G. A. T., *Nature* (1979), **277**, 289-391.
73. Gwadz, R. W. and Koontz, L. C., *Infect. Immun.* (1984), **44**, 137-145.
74. Kumar, N. and Carter, R., *Mol. Biochem. Parasitol.* (1984), **13**, 333-341.
75. Mendis, K., Udayama, P., Carter, R. and David, P. H., *J. Cell Biochem.* (1986), **10A (suppl.)**, 149-156.
76. Vermuelen, A. N., Ponnudurai, T., Beckers, P. J. A., Verhave, J. P., et al., *J. Exp. Med.* (1985), **162**, 1460-1476.
77. Rener, J., Graves, P. M., Carter, R., Williams, J. L., et al., *J. Exp. Med.* (1983), **158**, 976-980.
78. Graves, P. M., Carter, R., Burkot, T. R., Rener, J., et al., *Infect. Immun.* (1985), **48**, 611-619.

5. Immunotherapy

Alan S. Cross

5.1 Introduction

During the last 100 years considerable progress has been made in the evolution of our concepts of passive immunotherapy as well as in the development of preparations safe for human use; however, the proper role for such therapy in clinical medicine still needs to be defined.

By 1900 immune serum from various animal species had been used to treat pneumonia, tetanus, diphtheria and rabies. Human serum was first used in 1907 by Cenci for the modification of measles and later for mumps and pertussis [1]. Placental extracts that were prepared by ammonium sulfate precipitation [2, 3] were also used and may be considered the first immunoglobulins prepared for human use [3]. Placental material is still used as a source of immunoglobulin in some parts of the world.

The serious hypersensitivity reactions associated with animal serum proteins and the risk of viral hepatitis with convalescent human serum limited the use of serum therapy to life-threatening infections. In the 1920s attempts were made to separate by alcohol or acetone treatment the immune substances from the other constituents of animal serum. One such preparation, Huntoon's Antibody Solution, was administered intravenously to over 400 patients without the occurrence of anaphylaxis or serum sickness; however, pyrexia, cyanosis and dyspnea did occur and was implicated in the deaths of 3 patients in one study [4]. The introduction of antibiotics in the 1930s also decreased the demand for serum therapy [5]. During this time, however, the experimental basis for combination therapy with antimicrobials and hyperimmune animal serum was established [6, 7].

In 1936 Arne Tiselius separated serum proteins into 4 major fractions by electrophoresis and 2 years later, he and Kabat found immunoglobulin to be predominantly in the gamma electrophoretic fraction (see in [8]). The identification of the gamma fraction as rich in antibody could not be put to practical use, however, until Cohn and colleagues devised a procedure for recovering immunoglobulins from serum on a large scale. Cohn's group made feasible the large scale fractionation of serum proteins based on their differential solubility (precipitation) with various concentrations of ethanol under carefully controlled conditions of pH, temperature, protein concentration and ionic strength (see in [3, 9]). This process enriched and stabilized the gamma globulin from plasma at a relatively uniform antibody content while also denaturing most viruses [1]. Oncley et al. further refined the isolation procedures such that most gamma globulins are now made by a combination Cohn-Oncley procedure that can recover up to 60 % of the IgG or antibody activity of the starting plasma [3] (Fig. 5-1).

Cohn fraction II, the starting material for immunoglobulin preparations, contains IgG, with trace amounts of IgA and IgM and lacks most other serum proteins [11]. Such gamma globulin prepared from large (>500 donors) pools of donor plasma were used in the treatment of infectious diseases during World War II [11].

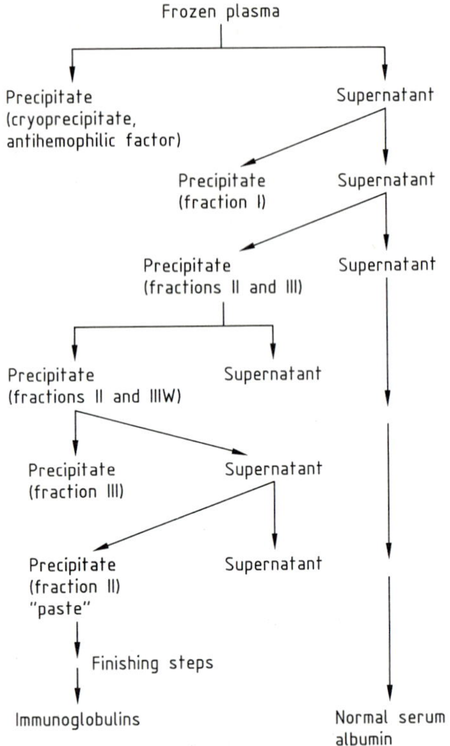

Fig. 5-1 Prepraration of immunoglobulin by Cohn-Oncley fractionation ("6/9 method"). Cohn fractionation by cold-alcohol procedures yields a fraction II precipitate or "paste". This is followed by applying the Oncley procedure to Cohn fraction II material to give immunoglobulin. The procedure is based on solubility differences that depend on ethanol concentration, ionic strenght, pH, temperature, and protein concentration. Precipitates are usually collected by centrifugation.

Shortly after the completion of World War II gamma globulin was shown to contain antibody titers adequate for the prevention or attenuation of measles [11], infectious hepatitis [12] and polio [13]. Since the report of hypogammaglobulinemia in 1952 by Bruton, and the demonstration by Janeway that ISG administered on a monthly basis decreased the incidence of infection [14], antibody replacement of this deficiency has been routine.

5.2 Properties and Preparation of Gamma Globulin

Five major isotypes of immunoglobulin have been defined. The functions of IgG, IgA and IgM are well described in the literature. IgE, which is involved both in allergy and in immune responses to parasites, and IgD, whose role in the circulation is still undefined, comprise the other two classes of antibody. Immunoglobulin G., at a serum concentration of 600-1200 mg/100 ml in adults, represents approximately 11-14 % of total serum proteins [8] and 80 % of serum antibody [15]. IgM and IgA have lower serum concentrations and shorter half-lives than IgG. The molecular weight has been estimated to be 145 000 [8], with 2.5 % by weight being carbohydrate that is associated with the H chain. The individual chains (2H and 2L) are held together by disulfide bonds and weak covalent forces [15].

IgG, which has a half-life in the normal circulation of approximately 25 days (35-40 days in patients with agammaglobulinemia) is synthesized by humans at a rate of 35 mg/kg/day in a 70 kg adult [15]. Its rate of synthesis is regulated by serum IgG levels such that the greater the serum immunoglobulin level the lower is the rate of synthesis.

Among the IgG isotype are 4 subclasses, based on 4 different types of gamma heavy chain genes, each with different properties (Tab. 5-1). IgG_1, which comprises approximately 2/3 of total IgG, binds to Fc receptors of neutrophils and mononuclear cells and to the first component of complement. This latter capability is believed to be based on the flexibility of the molecule in the hinge region. This is in turn dependent on the number of amino acids [16]. Antibodies to protein are predominantly of this subclass. Siber et al. noted that the antibody response to pneumococcal and Hemophilus polysaccharides may be related to the pre-immune levels of the IgG_2 subclass [17]. IgG_2, which is the last to reach mature levels in the neonate, activates the classical complement pathway poorly but can activate complement by the alternate pathway and represents 20-30 % of total IgG. It is more resistant to proteolysis than the other subtypes [15]. The remaining subclasses, IgG_3 and IgG_4, bind to Fc receptors of phagocytes and mast cells respectively and each comprise less than 10 % of total IgG [16]. IgG_3 has a short half-life (5-10 days). IgG_4 is unable to bind complement.

Tab. 5.1 Immunoglobulin G subclasses.

Property	IgG1	IgG2	IgG3	IgG4
% total IgG (adult)	60-70	20-30	5-10	< 5
Structure				
– mass (daltons)	146 000	146 000	170 000	146 000
– no. of interchain disulfide bonds	2	4	11	2
– no. of amino acids in hinge region	15	12	62	12
– kappa : lambda ratio of L chains	2.4	1.1	1.4	8.0
Catabolic rate (days)	21-23	20-23	7-8	21-23
Biologic activity				
- classical complement pathway activation (relative activity)	6	1	40	0
– Fc receptor binding				
mononuclear cells	2+	1+	2+	+ / –
neutrophils	2+	+/-	2+	1+
binding protein A	+	+	–	+

Adapted from [16].

Deficiencies in specific IgG subclasses are associated with increased risk of infection, particularly of the respiratory tract. Some patients with recurrent infections and low total IgG levels were found to have relatively greater decreases in specific IgG subclasses [18, 19]. Subsequently, Oxelius reported patients having normal total IgG, IgA and IgM levels, who completely lacked IgG2 and IgG4. These patients had severe upper airway infections [20]. Since then, patients with selective IgA and IgG2 deficiency and IgG4 deficiency have been described, all having increased susceptibility to respiratory tract infections (see [21]).

5.2.1 Immune Serum Globulin

Immune serum globulin (ISG) or gamma globulin is prepared from the plasma of pools of donors that contain >1000 individuals. This minimizes the differences among individual antibody levels to specific antigens, although regional differences have been found to specific antigens in such pools (e. g. diphtheria antitoxin-22).

ISG, which is usually prepared as a 16.5 % injectable solution (165 mg/ml) represents approximately a twenty to twenty-fivefold concentration of IgG found in plasma [3, 10]. Thus there is an effective dose of antibody in a relatively small volume [10]. Because of the viscosity of the preparation, the product can only be given intramuscularly or subcutaneously [10], usually through a large gauge needle (16-18 ga). It has been estimated that one gram of ISG has 4 x 10^{18} molecules with greater than 10^7 specificities [1]. The product, while highly stable at 4 °C, can still undergo proteolysis, presumably due to plasmin contamination which can ultimately break the IgG down to Fc and Fab fragments [3]. ISG may further contain blood group substances and antibody, IgA and IgG dimers. The presence of IgA can result in anaphylactic reactions in patients who lack IgA [3] (see below, "Adverse reactions").

Since he realized that high doses of antibody needed to be injected directly into the bloodstream, Cohn in 1948 gave 25-25 ml of ISG intravenously and saw no adverse effects (see in [3, 23]). Janeway, working with Cohn, repeated the experiment with a new preparation and induced severe reactions after only 2 ml. This reaction was later attributed to contamination of the preparation by staphylococcal enterotoxin [23]. The intravenous administration of ISG was repeated by Janeway in 1970 [3] and induced severe cardiovascular (tachycardia, arrhythmias, hypotension, severe chest pain), tachypneic and pyrogenic (fever, chills, malaise) reactions [10]. These adverse effects were attributed to the presence of high molecular weight immunoglobulin aggregates that form during the preparation of ISG and which may activate complement (anti-complementary activity) [24].

5.2.2 Immunoglobulin for Intravenous Use (IVIG)

Since the initial studies by Cohn and colleagues, there has been a need for a gamma globulin that could be administered by the intravenous route in order to provide greater patient comfort, increase its acceptability and administer larger quantities of antibody. This has been particularly true for patients with small muscle mass (children), insufficient skin surface (burns), at risk from uncontrollable bleeds (Wiskott-Aldrich or other bleeding diatheses) or those who need either large repeated doses (immunodeficient patients) or rapid onset of peak levels (intoxicated patients). With intramuscular administration there may also be degradation of ISG antibody at the local site of injection [25].

To avoid the problem of severe reactions that followed the intravenous infusion of ISG, methods of treating immunoglobulin were introduced to rid preparations of high molecular weight aggregates of immunoglobulin due to some denaturation that inevitably occurs during its preparation. These aggregates in ISG are believed to activate complement and to be the cause of the severe reactions [26]. While they could be removed by centrifugation, there was usually reaggregation. In addition, centrifugation was not practical on a large scale [27]. Consequently, chemical modification of the immunoglobulin was attempted to prevent the reaggregation.

Various methods of chemical modification have been tried. Pepsin was initially tried by Barandun since it had been used since the 1930s to "purify" animal sera. If allowed to proceed to completion, however, the pepsin treatment resulted in loss of Fc fragments with the loss of ability of the product to fix complement and a shortened serum half-life (thus making it less desirable for prophylaxis). Adjustment of the pH to 4.0 alone also prevented the immediate reaggregation, since it was known that the pH affects the aggregation of proteins in Cohn fraction II: at pH 7.4 aggregation was rapid and complete; lowering the pH delayed this occurrence. With storage, however, reaggregation occurred. The addition of pepsin at a much more dilute (1:100 000 instead of 1:100) concentration prevented the long term reaggregation while avoiding the loss of Fc-mediated function. With this procedure all the disulfide bonds were intact [31]. Other proteolytic enzymes, such as plasmin, also resulted in $F(ab)_2$ fragments [3]. Approximately 30-40 % of immunoglobulin resists plasmin treatment. Enzymatic treatment with pepsin or plasmin resulted in $F(ab')_2$ fragments [3] and Fc fragments, which had immunologic activity, such as the induction of prostaglandin E1 [28]. In addition, since the enzyme is not removed, its activity may have continued in the absence of lyophilization or the porcine pepsin may have induced antibody formation [26]. Acidification of immunoglobulin with HCl also prevented reaggregation [29]. Reaggregation was also prevented by cleavage of disulfide bonds. This may be done through reductive (dithiothreitol and iodoacetamide) or oxidative (sulfite and tetrathionite-3) methods. Alkylation and acylation has been accomplished with beta-propiolactone. In the United States, licensure was granted to a product that was reduced and alkylated, but that product has since been replaced by an unmodified preparation.

It is now appreciated that IVIG preparations that have been reduced and alkylated or otherwise modified may have impaired complement binding and altered subclass distribution [30], impaired opsonic activity *in vitro* [31], shortened serum half-life and decreased protective efficacy in experimental infection [32]. Consequently a new generation of IVIG preparations have been produced without modification ("native", or “intact”). These methods include treatment with pH 4, polyethylene glycol (PEG), ethanol precipitation, ultra- or diafiltration and/or use of ion exchange chromatography [24]. Currently, four unmodified products are licensed in the United States, all beginning with Cohn fraction II: one prepared by pH 4 treatment in the presence of trace amounts of pepsin, one prepared by ion exchange chromatography followed by ultrafiltration, a third by diafiltration, ultrafiltration and adjustment of pH to 4-4.5, and a fourth that utilizes PEG and ion exchange chromatography.

Commercially prepared IVIG is usually stabilized with a mono- or disaccharide, such as 10 % maltose [5] or glucose. The addition of maltose or other disaccharides to Cohn fraction II in place of the 0.3M glycine used in ISG decreases considerably the incidence of side effects that accompany the infusion of IVIG [3, 29], perhaps by minimizing precipitation or aggregation. This has been tested in a double blind, crossover study of 29 patients with hypogammaglobulinemia. Three of 29 patients had reactions to IVIG that contained maltose compared to 22/29 that had IVIG without maltose [33]. Maltose can cause a mild diuretic effect [34].

While in 1968 the only manufacturing requirements for commercial immunoglobulins were that they be 16.5 +/- 1.5 g of globulin/100 ml and greater than 90 % be of a defined electrophoretic mobility [35], ideal requirements published by the World Health Organization for current immunoglobulin products are more specific and include: preparation from pools of >1000 donors; free of kinins, plasmin and prekallikrein activity; low IgA content; as free as possible from aggregates; at least 90 % intact IgG without fragments; unmodified as possible so that it maintains opsonic, complement and other biologic activities; presence of all IgG subclasses; levels of antibody to at least 2 bacterial species or toxins and 2 viruses (to be ascertained by neutralization tests); at least 0.1 International Units of antibody to hepatitis B and a 1:1000 titer to hepatitis A [36]. In addition it recommended that manufacturers desribe any chemical modifications to the immunoglobulin and state the diluent. Finally a product can properly be identified as a hyperimmune immunoglobulin only if the antibody level is 5 times that of standard preparations.

There is no consensus on which laboratory test might predict the safety of IgG (contact activation, anticomplementary activity) [3]. In addition, one must now include among these requirements safety with regard to other virus transmission, particularly HIV, but also hepatitis B and non-A, non-B hepatitis, and IgG half-life [24].

5.3 Pharmacology

In contrast to the reasonably well-defined pharmacokinetics of ISG, the pharmacokinetics of IVIG are complicated by the variety of clinical conditions in which IVIG has been used as treatment.

Under the limited range of doses that one can administer intramuscularly, a dose of 100 mg/kg achieves a peak level in the blood at 24-48 hours and can elevate the baseline total IgG level by approximately 90 mg/100 ml blood [37]. The same dose of IVIG increased the total IgG approximately 200 mg/dl above baseline levels [37, 38]. There is a dose-dependent increase in serum IgG with increasing doses of IVIG such that at 500 mg/kg IgG, levels are increased by 975 mg/dl over pre-infusion levels [38]. Following these peak levels there is a bi-phasic decline in these levels post infusion with a rapid decline over days 3-7 at which time approx. 40 % of peak levels are present. This decline may occur even more rapidly in newborns. Thereafter, a slower decrease in the serum IgG occurs with baseline levels of IgG achieved in patients with hypogammaglobulinemia at approximately 21-28 days.

Changes in the serum levels are due to a number of mechanisms: the redistribution of the IgG in IVIG to other, non-vascular compartments, feedback inhibition of new IgG synthesis, accelerated catabolism of existing IgG and, in the case of disease, consumption by complex formation with microbial and nonmicrobial antigens.

In patients with primary immunodeficiency, numerous studies documented a serum half-life of approx. 21 days (see [39]). Half-lives for some commercially available IVIG preparations have ranged from 18-22 days in one study [40] to 31-32 days in another [41]. In the presence of infection, the serum half-life can be greatly shortened. Following the infusion of plasma to patients with agammaglobulinemia the half-life shortened from 32 days to 15 to 24 days [42]. In another patient with immunodeficiency, chronic malabsorption and fulminant sepsis, the serum half-life of the infused IVIG was 10.6 days [43]. The pharmacokinetics of antibody levels to specific antigens, as opposed to total IgG levels, are less defined. The administration of 400 mg/kg of a non-hyperimmune preparation elevated antibody to group B *Streptococcus* up to 80 % above preinfusion levels at 30 minutes; by day 2, however, the specific antibody was only a third above baseline levels [44].

5.4 Indications for Use

A wide variety of biologicals for passive immunotherapy are now available (Tab. .-2). ISG has been recommended for the short term prevention of disease when vaccines for active immunization are unavailable or when active immunization was not given before a disease exposure. In these instances ISG should be given before expected contact or early in the disease incubation, since it requires 4-7 days to achieve effective blood levels. In these situations active immunization is always preferable since passive therapy gives only short term protection. ISG is also used for antibody replacement in patients who lack adequate serum levels of immunoglobulin [2].

Tab. 5.2 Biologic products available for passive immunotherapy.

Standard immune globulin (16.5 %)

Standard immunoglobulin for intraveneous use (IVIG)

Hyperimmune globulins
- Anti-D immunoglobulin (Rhogam)
- Anti-lymphocyte immune globulin
- Diphtheria
- Hepatitis A
- Hepatitis B
- Measles
- Mumps
- Pertussis
- Polio
- Rabies
- Rubella
- Tetanus
- Tick borne encephalitis
- Vaccinia
- Varicella

Antitoxins
- Botulinus (equine)
- Diphtheria
- Gas gangrene (equine)

Investigational hyperimmune globulins
- Cytomegalovirus
- *P. aeruginosa*
- *H. influenzae* (type b), *Pneumococcus, Meningococcus* (combination)

There is no evidence, except in those instances enumerated below, that *standard immunoglobulin* is of any use in the prophylaxis of any disease in individuals without immune deficiency [23]. The efficacy of ISG for the prophylaxis of specific infections was established shortly after the widespread availability of ISG in the 1940s. These include:

Measles. The ability of convalescent serum to modify the course of measles was shown in 1907 [2]. ISG has been shown to prevent or attenuate the disease [10]; however, the introduction of active immunization with a measles vaccine in 1963 led to a significant decrease in the incidence of this disease in the United States and obviated the widespread need for ISG, except in a few specific patients. ISG is now recommended for use in infants <1 year of age or for those with immune deficiency within 6 days of acute exposure to a case of measles [36].

Rubella. Standard ISG is unreliable in the modification of rubella [2, 4, 45]. High titers of antibody are needed [33]. Nevertheless, the use of ISG is considered optional for women exposed to the disease during early pregnancy [36].

Hepatitis. Stokes and Neefe showed that ISG could prevent or modify the course of hepatitis A [2, 3, 12]. Krugman however, found ISG modified, but could not prevent this disease in his studies at Willowbrook [45]. The dose for hepatitis A is 0.02 ml/kg [3]. A hyperimmune antibody preparation for hepatitis A is available commercially.

In the case of hepatitis B, ISG is not recommended. Rather, hyperimmune globulin is given after mucosal or percutaneous exposure (including sexual contact) to an antigen positive individual [3]. It is also recommended for newborns of antigen positive mothers [36]. While Grossmann et al. [46] found ISG to decrease the incidence of post-transfusion hepatitis, its use for non-A, non-B hepatitis is currently considered optional [36].

Polio. The efficacy of ISG, if given early, to modify the paralytic complications of polio was shown in the late 1940s [2, 13].

Prevention of Infection in Patients With Hypogammaglobulinemia. A dose of 100 mg/kg (IM) given every 3-4 weeks, the currently recommended dose of ISG, will maintain a level of circulating IgG above 200 mg/ml [3]. This level will confer protection against a wide variety of infections [9]. This recommendation is based on a study by the British Medical Research Council conducted between 1956-1966 on 176 patients who, following a loading dose of 200-300 mg/kg to raise the serum IgG to >2 g/l, were randomized into a regimen of 25 or 50 mg/kg/week (no placebo controls were given since Janeway already demonstrated the efficacy of ISG to prevent infection in these patients). In this study no optimal regimen was identified, due in part to the similarity of the two doses and the heterogeneity of the patient population [47]. This study therefore established only a minimum dose. While serum IgG levels at this dose of ISG rarely rise to the normal range [48], there appears to be no need to totally replace the IgG to prevent infection [49]. While the optimal dose has not yet been established, one study did compare the prophylactic efficacy of different doses of ISG. A dose of 200 mg/kg/month was found superior to 100 mg/kg; however most patients did not tolerate more than the 100 mg/kg/month [33]. Two other studies also showed that higher doses of ISG decreased the incidence of acute infections [1]. Since there may be individual variations in the levels of IgG following specific doses, individualization of doses for patients with hypogammaglobulinemia has been suggested with changes in either dose or frequency [48]. IVIG has now clearly been shown to be effective in the prevention of infection in patients with hypogammaglobulinemia [30]. It has also been shown to be effective in the treatment of chronic infection in such patients who developed sinopulmonary infection despite ISG maintenance therapy [25].

In addition to patients with primary hypogammaglobulinemia, it is also recommended to administer immunoglobulin to patients with other conditions that result in diminished immunoglobulin levels, such as those with Wiskott-Aldrich syndrome, and common variable immunodeficiency. In addition, patients with IgG subclass deficiencies, even in the presence of normal total IgG levels, should receive immunoglobulin, since they are susceptible to severe, recurrent pyogenic infections of the respiratory tract.

High titered preparations of ISG (hyperimmune) prepared from the plasma of patients recently recovered from the disease or from those with known high titers from previous vaccination or natural infection have been prepared for use in:

Tetanus.

Varicella. The efficacy of standard ISG in the prophylaxis of this disease is not well-established [2, 45]. Use of the hyperimmune product, however, is indicated in individuals who have never had chicken pox, who are exposed to acute cases and belong to a high risk group such as newborns or immunocompromised patients, and pregnant women [36].

Rabies. Hyperimmune globulin is recommended in addition to active immunization following exposure to a possible or proven case of rabies [36]. There is no controlled trial that demonstrates the efficacy of hyperimmune globulin, but active and passive immunization against rabies has been shown to be superior to active immunization alone [3].

Mumps. ISG has no efficacy in the modification of this disease, but hyperimmune has [10].

Polio.

Pertussis. Hyperimmune globulin modifies the disease. For example, 2.5 ml of hyperimmune anti-pertussis gamma globulin with a follow-up dose at 5-7 days led to a 75 % reduction in disease among non-immune, exposed individuals [10]. This has been superseded by the use of antibiotics [22].

Vaccinia. The hyperimmune globulin is used for prophylaxis against smallpox and for treatment of the dermal complications of vaccination [10].

Diphtheria [9].

Rho(D) immune globulin. This hyperimmune globulin is recommended for Rh negative mothers who deliver Rh positive infants [36].

Globulins with high titers to CMV and *Pseudomonas aeruginosa* are currently being tested.

5.5 Clinical Studies

5.5.1 Immune Serum Globulin (ISG)

Prophylaxis. Having evaluated the data available in 1980, a committee of the WHO observed that it was "inappropriate" to use standard immunoglobulin for the prevention of infection in premature infants, during the physiologic hypogammaglobulinemia of infancy or for malnutrition. Its use is contraindicated in patients with selective IgA deficiency because of the risk of anaphylaxis (see below, "Adverse reactions" [36]). Previous attempts in the 1960s to prophylax infection with ISG in a variety of clinical situations showed no efficacy [50, 51]. ISG given prophylactically to patients with multiple myeloma at 100 mg/kg did not decrease the incidence of infections [52]. ISG, at a dose of 0.15-0.4 ml per pound given every 3 or 6 months was unable to prevent upper or lower respiratory tract infections in 113 children or 357 institutionalized, elderly adults; however, a significant decrease was seen in the incidence of mumps in children and fevers of unknown origin in adults [53].

Its use in the prevention of infection in burned patients has yielded conflicting data [2]. In a prospective, randomized study, Kefalides et al. administered plasma, ISG or saline at a dose of 1 ml/kg intramuscularly on admission and on days 3 and 5 to Peruvian children who suffered burns over at least 10 % of their body surface area in an attempt to prevent septic death (mostly from *P. aeruginosa*). There was a 41 % incidence of septicemia and 15 % mortality in control patients compared to a 21 % incidence of septicemia and 6 % mortality among those who received either plasma or ISG [54]. In an attempt to confirm these findings, Stone et al. gave ISG at a dose of 2.0-0.6 ml/kg every 3d day to 100 patients with burns admitted to Grady Hospital. They observed no beneficial effect from such treatment on either the rate of septicemia or mortality [55]. More recently, patients admitted to a burn unit in India were randomized into groups that received active immunization against *P. aeruginosa* (78 patients), passive immunization with a cold ethanol precipitate of plasma from normal immunized volunteers [31], both immunologic treatments [28] or neither [42]. In children, but not adults, there was a significant reduction of mortality from 21 % (9/42 to 0/18) following a dose of just over 20 mg protein a day for three days. There was a decrease in the incidence of not only *P. aeruginosa*, but also other Gram-negative bacilli among those treated immunologically [56].

The ability of ISG to prevent infections has been most extensively studied in high risk, premature infants (Tab. 5-3). This population has a well-documented physiological hypogammaglobulinemia that exposes them to a high incidence of bacterial infection [57]. The more premature the infant the lower the IgG-level, since most of the transplacental transfer of IgG occurs during the last 6 weeks of gestation [50]. Children do not attain adult levels of immunoglobulin until 2 years of age. In two studies that gave between 0.5 ml/kg to 3 ml/kg of ISG no prophylactic effect was observed in the small numbers of patients in each study [51, 58], although there was a suggestion that the high dose regimen may have had a beneficial effect. In each case, the investigators noted they were restricted to small doses.

Tab. 5-3 Use of ISG and IVIG in prophylaxis of infection in neonates.

Study	Group studied (Dose)	Results	Immunoglobulin	No Immunoglobulin (control)	Comments
		Immune Serum Globulin (ISG)			
Steen [58]	1000-2000 g (0.5 ml/kgq 2 wks x 4 mos)	severe infxn	2/10	2/10	open study
		mild infxn	4/10	4/10	
Amer et al. [51]	"premature infants" (3 ml/kg x 1)	deaths	1/92	6/68	113 infants left study; trends not statistically significant
		infxn-free	39/92	8/92	
		severe infxn	14/92	15/92	
Conway et al. [60]	under 32 wks	deaths	0/59	3/61	3 episodes of NEC all in control
		infxn-free	46/59	45/61	
		bacteremia	18/59	28/61	
		total infxns	22/59	40/61	
Santosham et al. [59]	infants (0.5 ml/kg; at 2,6 & 10 mos)	infxn D1-90	0/353	11/350	hyperimmune v. Pn & Hib bacteremia and meningitis endpoints
		after D90	11/353	10/350	
		Intravenous Immune Globulin (IVIG)			
Sidiropoulos et al. [61]	women with chorioamnionitis 27-36 wks ofgestation (24 g/day; for 5 days)	infxn low dose	3/9	6/16	all neonates under 32 wks infected; no transplacenta-transfer of IgG.
		infxn high dose	0/7	00	
Chirico et al. [50]	under 1500g (0.5 mg/kg/wk; for 4 weeks)	total infxns	22/43	31/40	no differences if over 1500g
		deaths	1/43	6/43	
Haque et al. [62]	under 1500 g (120 mg/kg)	infxn	2/50	8/50	High bachground rates
Haque et al. [63]	under 37 wks	infxn	21/30	23/30	IgM-enriched preparation
		deaths	4/30	1/30	
Stabile et al. [64]	under 34 wks or 1500g (500mg/kg; days 1,2,3,7,14,21,28)	infxn	5/40	3/40	infxns all bacteremia or meningitis; no differences
		deaths	5/40	3/40	

NB: Infxn, infection; NEC,, necrotizing enterocolitis; Pn, pneumococcal; Hib, Hemophilus influenzae type b; wk(s), week(s); mos, months.

Certain subpopulations of children, such as native American Indians and Eskimos, are at particularly high risk of acquiring serious infection with encapsulated bacteria. Since previous studies failed to show a beneficial prophylactic effect for many types of infection with standard ISG preparations, Santosham et al. randomized 703 Apache infants into receiving saline at a dose of 0.5 ml/kg intramuscularly at 2, 6 and 10 months of age or ISG made hyperimmune to polysaccharide antigens by immunizing volunteers with licensed vaccines against *Pneumococcus*, *H. influenzae* and *Meningococcus*. There was a significant reduction in the incidence of systemic disease caused by *H. influenzae* and *Pneumococcus* during the first 6 months of follow up as well as a significant decrease in the incidence of bacteremia [59].

Treatment. While there is data that ISG is active in bacterial infections in animal models [22, 65] and may be synergistic with antibiotics [6, 7, 66], Schless and Harrell [22] and others, observed that in 1968 there was little evidence for its therapeutic efficacy in established infection in humans and suggested the need for a controlled clinical trial of ISG in the *treatment* of systemic infection in patients that were not deficient in antibody [22]. Indeed, it has been speculated that since most functionally-active antibody to Gram-negative bacteria was IgM and not the IgG found in ISG, that there would be little benefit expected [9]. ISG has been known to have activity against a wide variety of human pathogens in animal models of infection [22]. When used with antimicrobial agents, ISG has been shown to have possible benefit in both experimental infection with a wide variety of organisms [66, 67] and in clinical infection in man [6, 7, 68, 69]. This latter report described a series of cases, however, where ISG given with antibiotics appeared to clear the infections in some patients who had earlier failed when either modality was given alone. No alteration in serum bactericidal activity was noted in those patients who recovered from infection [68].

In 1964 Bodey administered daily large doses (10 ml/m^2 body surface) of ISG intravenously for 10 days to 46 patients who had leukemia and fever. While no benefit was found for patients who received the ISG in addition to antibiotics (compared to antibiotics alone), the intravenous ISG was well tolerated [70]. The administration of ISG to shorten the course of infection in children <2 years of age admitted to the hospital was ineffective [71].

5.5.2 Plasma and Other Blood Products

While the use of plasma and other blood products is considered impractical for large scale, regular clinical use (both for production and safety reasons), a number of studies have shown that the passive immunotherapy may provide some efficacy in the prophylaxis and treatment of infections in man.

Plasma has been used to treat infections, particularly those caused by *Pseudomonas* [54, 72]. In the latter study, plasma therapy was superior to treatment with ISG in the prevention of infection among patients who suffered $> 30\%$ burns. Similar observations were made during experimental infection [73]. One possible explanation for the efficacy of plasma is the inclusion of immunoglobulins G, A and M. This may improve the distribution of antibodies at different anatomic sites and, since the different isotypes have functional differences, the antibacterial activity. In addition, natural antibodies against Gram-negative bacilli have been thought to be predominantly of the IgM isotype. Plasma infusions do carry the risk of transmitting hepatitis, since there is no manufacturing process for plasma that inactivates the virus as is the case with the preparation of ISG.

Although the defective neonatal opsonic response was shown to be partially correctable with gamma globulin [74], the ability of passively administered opsonins to prevent infection was first suggested in a study in which fresh whole blood was administered for the purpose of preventing group B streptococcal sepsis. All 9 infants transfused with blood having antibody to GBS lived versus 3/6 transfused with blood having undetectable antibody titers. Protection was correlated with opsonic antibody titers in the infants' blood and with having greater than 40 % of their blood volume replaced [75].

In a recent study, the passive administration of post-immune serum from individuals immunized with the J5 mutant of *Escherichia coli* O111:B4 to elicit antibodies to widely shared core epitopes in the LPS of Gram-negative bacilli was shown to decrease the incidence of death from endotoxic shock, as well as the need for pressor therapy in patients in profound shock compared to patients who had received pre-immune plasma. However this protection did not correlate with antibody to the core epitopes. Thus it is not clear whether the protection was even conferred by antibody [76]. In a follow-up randomized, controlled and prospective study, the prophylactic administration of plasma taken from donors after immunization with the J5 mutant bacteria appeared to significantly prevent shock and death from Gram-negative infections in patients admitted to a surgical intensive care unit, particularly those with abdominal surgery. Such treatment had no effect on infection rate, however [77]. In both studies the presumed protective moiety in the plasma and serum was antibody to the toxic effects of endotoxin, although this was not shown directly. In any case, for this to be a practical therapy the active protective portion of the postimmune product must be able to be mass produced in a standardized, safe preparation (e. g. made into an IVIG from a large pool of donors immunized with the J5 vaccine or into a monoclonal antibody preparation). Attempts to show a protective effect from an IVIG prepared from immunized donors have been unsuccessful to date [78]. Nevertheless, monoclonal antibody preparations directed toward a J5 epitope are currently being evaluated in human volunteers.

Further efforts in the use of passive immunotherapy have also focused on septic shock. The rapid infusion of large volumes of freeze dried human plasma from units of blood having greater than 40 mg/ml of antibody to a mixture of O antigens resulted in a nearly 7-fold decrease in mortality in South African women treated in an obstetrical/gynecologic ward for septic shock [79]. Use of equine plasma similarly screened for anti-lipopolysaccharide antibodies has been used routinely in veterinary practice in that country [80]. Finally, a murine monoclonal antibody directed against tumor necrosis factor, a cytokine believed to be a principal mediator of septic shock, has been administered to 14 patients in septic shock [81].

5.5.3 IVIG

In studies examining the prophylactic or therapeutic efficacy of ISG, the possibility that higher doses of standard immunoglobulin might prove to be effective was a recurring theme. With the availability of IVIG it was now possible to administer larger volumes of immunoglobulin directly into the bloodstream, achieve increased serum levels of IgG more promptly and, especially in the case of children, with less pain. In addition, with the ability to screen large numbers of samples for antibody levels or to immunize volunteers with an increasing number of vaccines, there has been an enlarging literature examining the efficacy of passive immunotherapy, particularly with hyperimmune preparations, in the treatment and prophylaxis of infectious diseases.

5.5.3.1 Viral Infection

Prophylaxis. Since CMV is such a frequent cause of infection in patients undergoing organ transplantation, and since there is a lack of effective antiviral therapy, there has been considerable interest in the use of IVIG that is hyperimmune in CMV antibody in both the prophylaxis and treatment of CMV infection. Such CMV-IVIG was shown to decrease the attack rate of symptomatic CMV infection among 59 CMV-negative patients who received kidneys from CMV antibody-positive donors from 60 to 21 % when given as prophylaxis to renal transplant patients at a total dose of 550 mg/kg during the first 4 months post transplantation [82]. This treatment also decreased the incidence of fungal and parasitic infection. Condie and O'Reilly also have shown efficacy of CMV-IVIG in the prevention of mortality and interstitial pneumonia from CMV for 120 days when given at 200 mg/kg at 25, 50 and 75 days post transplantation in the prevention of CMV in a small group of leukemic patients who underwent bone marrow transplantation (BMT) [83]. In a random, controlled trial, use of non-immune IVIG that had a final ELISA titer of 1:6400 against CMV at a dose of 20 ml/kg/week did not decrease the incidence of CMV seroconversion compared to controls when given as prophylaxis to BMT patients [84]; however, there was a decrease in the incidence of symptoms and in interstitial pneumonia. CMV-IVIG prophylaxis was shown to prevent interstitial pneumonia but not the acquisition of infection in patients with bone marrow transplant [85]. In contrast, Bowden et al. found that CMV-IVIG when given to 97 patients who were negative for CMV before BMT had no effect on either the prevention of new disease or the amelioration of established disease [86].

Treatment. Immune globulin has been used sporadically in the treatment of viral disease. Reed et al. were unable to demonstrate efficacy or high-titered IVIG from screened donors when given at 400 ml/kg on days 1, 2, 7 and every week thereafter in the treatment of BMT patients with documented CMV infection [87]. When high doses of IVIG hyperimmune to CMV was given in combination with ganciclovir (9-1,3 dihydroxy-2-propoxymethylguanine), however, to patients who acquired CMV pneumonitis after BMT, a highly significant response was noted at 10 months of follow-up compared to patients treated with either modality alone [88]. These data were confirmed in a second study that utilized historical controls [89] and in experimental infection models. The use of polyvalent IVIG that was not hyperimmune to CMV did not have a therapeutic benefit for renal transplantation patients infected with CMV [90]. Thus, as in the case of bacteria (see below), the combination of IVIG and antimicrobial agents can be synergistic. IVIG has been shown to alter the course of echovirus encephalitis infection in 3 patients with hypogammaglobulinemia. In two of these patients no benefit occurred from giving the IVIG intravenously; however, intraventricular administration of the IVIG through an Ommaya reservoir resulted in sterile cultures and clinical cures at 28 and 16 months after therapy [91, 92]. One patient suffered a relapse 7 months after therapy [92]. The use of IVIG was unable to alter the lethal course of polymyositis secondary to echovirus in another patient with hypogammaglobulinemia [93]. IVIG has also been used experimentally in the treatment of herpes infection in mice [94].

5.5.3.2 Bacterial Infection

Prophylaxis. Earlier data with ISG in both experimental bacterial infection in animals and in clinical infection in man indicated that in some cases, such as hypogammaglobulinemia, exogenous standard gamma globulin could prevent the acquisition of serious bacterial infection. Similar studies with IVIG have established the efficacy of these preparations [30]. A number of studies compared ISG with IVIG, but not in a randomized, blinded fashion. It appears that one must give at least 150 mg/kg of IVIG every 4 weeks to achieve levels that prevent infection.

Since earlier investigators believed that if it were possible to give larger doses of ISG it might be possible to demonstrate efficacy in the prevention of bacterial infection in high risk neonates, it is not surprising that similar studies have now been reported with IVIG (Tab. 5.3). In one nursery where there was a high rate of infection, IVIG was given at a dose of 120 mg/kg within 2 hrs of birth to preterm, low birthweight neonates. Infections were observed in 8/50 infants not receiving IVIG but in only 2/50 treated patients [62]. There was also a significant decrease in mortality among treated infants. A second dose of IVIG at 8 days, however, conferred no advantage. This same group later reported that an IVIG preparation enriched in IgM antibody (Pentaglobin, IgM was 12 % of total immunoglobulin) significantly improved mortality from 6/30 (20 %) to 1/30 (3.3 %) in this same setting of high background mortality rates in their neonatal unit. Chirico and associates administered 0.5 mg/kg/wk for 4 weeks in a controlled fashion to 133 neonates at high risk of acquiring infection. Prophylaxis with IVIG was significantly better in preventing infection and death only in the subpopulation that weighed less than 1500 grams and had a gestational age of less than 34 weeks, but was no better than untreated controls in those neonates weighing greater than 1500 g despite the use of mechanical ventilation and other procedures common to intensive care [50]. Stabile and colleagues administered IVIG (at a dose of 500 mg/kg on days 1,2,3,7,14,21 and 28 of life) to 46 premature newborns, all weighing <1500 g and <34 weeks of age. In this study, there was no difference between IVIG-treated infants and 40 untreated controls in incidence of sepsis or mortality [64]. In another study to assess the possible efficacy of prophylaxis of bacterial infection of high risk neonates, antibiotics were given either alone or with IVIG to women pregnant 27-36 weeks who had chorioamnionitis. Only high dose IVIG (24 g/day for 5 days) given after the 32nd

week of pregnancy prevented infection in the delivered babies. All neonates born before 32 weeks and 30-40 % of babies of mothers who received 12 g/day for 5 days became infected [61]. These investigators concluded that little transplacental transfer of IgG occurred before the 32nd week of gestation.

Data for the use of standard IVIG for the prevention of bacterial infection of patients who do not have hypogammaglobulinemia is limited. This may be due in part to the need of high levels of specific antibody that may not be found in standard, non-immune IVIG, despite the ability to deliver larger amounts of IVIG than was the case with ISG. Such hyperimmune products have been shown to be effective in the prevention of specific infections in experimental models (see above, under ISG and below). The administration of non-immune IVIG at 1000 mg/kg before BMT and weekly for 17 weeks thereafter had no effect on the acquisition of either bacterial or fungal infection [76]. A study evaluating IVIG for the prophylaxis of bacterial infection in patients with chronic lymphocytic leukemia, a condition which may be complicated by hypogammaglobulinemia, has shown that such treatment at the end of a year's treatment, can decrease the incidence of mild infections (infections that could be treated with oral antimicrobial agents), but did not alter the risk of acquiring severe infections [96]. The IVIG was administered at 400 mg/kg every week for one year.

Patients with HIV infection are now recognized as having a dysfunction in their humoral immune system which includes both a decreased antibody response to bacterial antigens and an altered distribution of IgG subclasses [97]. Unlike adults who tend to acquire opportunistic infections, young children and particularly infants with these diagnosis, often resemble patients with primary humoral immunodeficiency and tend to become ill with bacterial infections. Consequently prophylaxis with monthly IVIG has been used in the management of these patients. In one pilot study, a decreased incidence in episodes of fever and bacteremia was noted. This was accompanied by clinical improvement and prolongation of life, as well as an improvement in other immunologic parameters [97]. In a 37 month old child with the acquired immunodeficiency syndrome (AIDS) given monthly IVIG to prevent his recurrent episodes of pneumococcal bacteremia, an increase in IgG_2 antibody, increase in antibody to 12 pneumococcal serotypes and prevention of subsequent episodes of bacteremia were observed [98]. On the basis of these preliminary data, the use of IVIG prophylaxis has been advocated by some investigators [97], although a well-controlled, prospective study has yet to be done. Periodic IVIG decreased lactic dehydrogenase activity, proposed as an indicator of pulmonary interstitial inflammation, in 16 adults and 17 children with HIV infection [99].

Treatment. Attempts to demonstrate a significant effect in the therapy of infections with IVIG have been much less successful. This may in part be attributable to the shorter half-life of IVIG in the blood during infection [48, 65]. Sideropoulos et al. reported that the addition of IVIG to standard regimens of antibiotics decreased the mortality from documented bacteremia, particularly among preterm infants. The number of subjects studied was too small for statistical analysis, however [100]. The use of IVIG in the absence of a specific pathogen has shown marginal improvement in some clinical parameters. The addition of IVIG to antibiotics for children with leukemia, fever and neutropenia resulted in a shorter duration of fever than patients receiving antibiotics alone, but no change in duration of neutropenia or hospitalization [101].

Patients with cystic fibrosis hospitalized for acute pulmonary exacerbations demonstrated improved pulmonary function when compared to patients receiving standard treatment alone [102]. The benefit in each of these studies might not be sufficient to justify routine IVIG use in similar situations.

In adults, there are little data that establish the use of IVIG in the treatment of bacterial infections. This may be due in part to the need for high levels of antibody specific for the invading organism (rather than simply high levels of non-specific antibody) as well as the need for prompt initiation of therapy. In the report by Shigeoka et al. the provision of exogenous opsonins required replacement of greater than 40 % of total blood volume [75]. In most of the experimental studies with hyperimmune IVIG little benefit from exogenous immunoglobulin can be shown if given 8 hrs after infection (see below, also [65]). In clinical medicine, however, it is often difficult to identify the time of onset of infection.

Experimental. Numerous studies have demonstrated the efficacy of hyperimmune IVIG in the prophylaxis and, if used early after infection, the treatment of bacterial infections. Over 45 years ago Alexander showed that the combination of sulfa and animal hyperimmune sera was more effective in reducing mortality (a 30-90 fold increase in LD50) than either agent alone [6, 7]. Recently a number of studies have demonstrated the efficacy of IVIG in both the prevention and treatment of experimental infection with *H. influenzae* in neonatal rat models [103], *E. coli* [104] and *Klebsiella* [105] in mouse models and *P. aeruginosa* in neutropenic and burned rodent models [106, 107]. IVIG hyperimmune to group B streptococcal surface antigens can prevent and treat serious bacteremia in experimental infection in monkeys [108]. Preparations of IVIG have significant titers of antibody that can neutralize Shiga 1 and Shiga-like bacterial toxins that may be associated with the hemolytic-uremic syndrome. Such anticytotoxin-neutralizing antibody may find use in the treatment of this intoxication in children [109].

5.6 Immunoglobulins Administered Orally

In addition to their use parenterally, immunoglobulin preparations have also been administered orally to either prevent of modify diseases whose primary site of entry and action is the gastrointestinal tract. Having previously demonstrated that ISG preparations retain their opsonic activity in the gastrointestinal tract of low birth weight infants, Kim et al. fed modified ISG with a high antibody level against type III group B *Streptococcus* before oral challenge with the homologus organism. Animals treated in this way had a significiantly lower rate of both gastrointestinal colonization and systemic disease than controls who received albumin. This protective effect of the ISG was felt to be at the mucosal level [110]. In a study of low birth weight infants at risk of acquiring necrotizing enterocolitis (NEC), IgA-IgG (73 % IgA, 26 % IgG) made from Cohn fraction II of normal human serum prevented the development of NEC [111]. This preparation, with high levels of antibody to both common viral and bacterial pathogens, resulted in intact IgA and IgG in the stool of treated infants, with no evidence of absorption into the serum. A novel approach to passive immunotherapy uses immunoglobulin concentrates from the colostrum of cows to treat infantile diarrhea caused by rotavirus, enteropathogenic *E. coli* and *Cryptosporidium* [112]. This concept has been recently extended to travelers' diarrhea. Volunteers who received milk immunoglobulins prepared from the colostrum of cows immunized with several enterotoxigenic *E. coli* serotypes, heat-labile enterotoxin and cholera toxin, had highly significant protection upon challenge with enterotoxigenic *E. coli* [113]. Since the immunoglobulin concentrate did not prevent recovery of the strain from the stool, its protective effect may have been due to its neutralizing effect on the toxin.

5.7 Diagnostic Use of IVIG

Patients with occult infection often require non-invasive radiologic tests in an attempt to locate a hidden site of infection toward which further diagnostic or therapeutic interventions may be directed. A gallium scan requires days to complete and the regular excretion through the gastrointestinal tract may obscure an infected site at that location. Similarly, scanning a patient with indium-labelled neutrophils requires the removal of blood from the patient, isolation and radiolabelling of the neutrophils followed by their reinfusion. Recently, Rubin et al. have demonstrated that the infusion of radiolabelled commercial IVIG can lead to the diagnosis of focal sites of inflammation and some cancers more quickly, more cheaply and with little background interference [114]. Since the localization of the IVIG is not due to specific immunologic properties of the IgG, but rather to nonimmunologic interactions with inflammatory cells or products of inflammation, this technique does not rely on the presence of type specific antibody toward a putative microorganism. Further experience with this technique seems warranted.

5.8 Uses of IVIG in Non-infectious Diseases

In 1981 it was reported that a patient who received IVIG for hypogammaglobulinemia also recovered from bleeding secondary to a coincidental thrombocytopenia following the infusion [115]. Following this serendipitous observation this group demonstrated experimentally that high dose IVIG could indeed reverse thrombocytopenia in the absence of hypogammaglobulinemia and that a regimen of 400 mg/kg/day for 5 days was effective treatment for ITP [116]. In this latter study Imbach and colleagues compared the use of IVIG to oral steroids in 108 children with ITP. Among those who responded rapidly to treatment (62 % of the 108), IVIG was as efficacious as steroids; however among the slower responders those randomized to the IVIG treatment responded better.

This was accompanied by a 2-fold increase in serum IgG. IgM levels rose under both treatment regimens. Fehr et al. observed in 4 adults that such a regimen induced a marked, transient defect in the reticuloendothelial (RE) clearance mechanism and postulated that perhaps the IVIG reduced the clearance of antibody-coated platelets via an Fc-mediated mechanism [117]. Other putative mechanisms have been invoked to explain this clinical response (see below). The dosage regimen used in Imbach's study, 400 mg/kg/day for 5 days (total of 2 g/kg) has been used in many of the other studies of uses of IVIG in non-infectious diseases. In one study 800-1000 mg/kg was given as a single infusion to 11 children with ITP with similar results and no reported untoward effects [118].

Since these original reports, IVIG has been used in the treatment of immunologically-mediated blood disorders in both pediatric and adult populations. These have included autoimmune hemolytic anemia [119, 120], autoimmune neutropenia [121], post-transfusion purpura [112], ITP in adults [123, 124], chronic ITP in both adults and children [125, 126], thrombocytopenia secondary to alloimmunization in leukemic patients receiving platelet transfusions, who became refractory to subsequent platelet transfusions [127], thrombocytopenia secondary to transplacental passage of anti-platelet antibodies [128] as well as in the ITP of pregnancy [129], antibody-mediated red cell aplasia {130], during pregnancy in women with severe Rh immunization [131] and in conjunction with cyclophosphamide, in the treatment of antibody to factor VIII in hemophilia [132]. The experience with IVIG for ITP has not been uniformly successful however [133].

In addition to these hematologic disorders, two large trials have been conducted in patients with Kawasaki's disease both of which compared the use of aspirin alone to that of aspirin and IVIG at 400 mg/kg/day for 4 and 3 days [134, 135]. One of these studies found that the incidence of coronary artery disease detected by 2-dimensional echocardiography significantly fell from 23 % in the aspirin-alone-group to 8 % in the aspirin-plus-IVIG-group [134]. In the other study as well, IVIG reduced the fever and the incidence of coronary artery disease [135]. IVIG suppressed the T and B cell activation characteristic of patients with this disease and decreased the level of spontaneous immunoglobulin synthesis *in vitro* [136].

High dose immunoglobulin treatment has also been used in patients with Felty's syndrome [137], myasthenia gravis {138], epilepsy [139] and multiple sclerosis [140]. In the latter study one-third of patients actually worsened with IVIG therapy.

In one interesting study, placentally derived immunoglobulin was administered to patients with severe rheumatoid arthritis (RA) since it was known that the symptoms of some patients with RA improved during pregnancy {141]. None of 5 control patients given IVIG derived from plasma improved whereas 3/5 improved under the placentally derived globulin. An anti-HLA-DR antibody in the placental preparation was presumed to be a possible mechanism for this improvement.

Experimental. The basis for the use of IVIG in non-infectious illnesses is not known. Many immunologic mechanisms have been invoked to explain the beneficial effects of IVIG and these usually involve an enlarging literature that demonstrates IVIG itself to be a potent immune modulator. The role of the Fc portion of the molecule in this activity is still a subject of active investigation.

Initially it was proposed that the Fc receptors in the RE system become saturated by the high dose IVIG and this resulted in a decreased clearance of IgG-coated particles via competitive inhibition [119, 142]. This is consistent with studies in patients in which radiolabelled, autologous erythrocytes were cleared more slowly after IVIG infusion than before [117, 125]. In one study such treatment was found to alter Fc receptor affinity, not receptor number [143]. Other mechanisms invoked include a decreased synthesis in autoantibodies [144], the clearance of persistent, occult viral infections that have been hypothesized to initiate some of these diseases [93, 144] as well as the protection of platelets or megakaryocytes from antiplatelet antibodies [144], anti-idiotypic suppression of antibody synthesis [139, 145] and anti-Fc receptor blocking, anti-lymphocyte antibody [146]. In support of one of these hypotheses, IVIG was shown to correct pure red cell aplasia that was ultimately found to be associated with a persistant (10 years) parvovirus B19 infection [147]. IVIG has also been shown to inhibit the MLC reaction, the cytotoxicity of NK cells [124, 148], ADCC and PHA stimulation of lymphocytes [139], and induce lymphocytopenia [149]. In 5 patients who received IVIG for myasthenia gravis, a selective effect in decreasing the ratio of helper to suppressor T cells was observed [150].

In some studies, however, patients with ITP responded to IVIG without demonstrable alteration in Fc-receptor mediated clearance [144]. Recent data suggest that the improvement observed in patients who respond to IVIG when given for ITP is not due to a reduction in platelet-reactive autoantibodies [151]. In addition, preincubation of erythrocytes in IVIG failed to inhibit the phagocytosis of sensitized erythrocytes by cultured macrophages [152]. Thus there may be multiple mechanisms by which IVIG may lead to improvement in such patients.

It is now clear that IVIG is quite potent both *in vitro* and *in vivo* in the modulation of antibody production. It inhibits lectin-driven B cell differentiation *in vitro* [153, 154] and immunoglobulin production by peripheral blood mononuclear cells stimulated with pokeweed mitogen [154]. For these effects the Fc portion of immunoglobulin must be present [153, 154]. In these studies the Fc portion alone was 100-fold more effective than the intact IgG. The observation that IgM antibody rises after IVIG infusion has raised the possibility that some immunoglobulin-producing cell populations may be stimulated [125]. Interestingly, the monthly administration of ISG to premature infants during the first year of life resulted in a significantly lower level of immunoglobulin compared to the control group [51, 155].

In adults with ITP, the infusion of 400 mg/kg led to a decrease in T4 and elevation in T8 lymphocytes (and decrease in T4/T8 ratio) [123]. Similarly, the administration of IVIG to patients with hypogammaglobulinemia led to increased suppressor T cell activity, decreased total T cells and a significant decrease in T4/T8 ratio [156]. There was also a decrease in lectin-induced immunoglobulin synthesis *in vitro* (which may correspond to a decrease in polyclonal antibody synthesis). In one study in which IVIG corrected antibody-mediated red cell aplasia, the activity of the cytotoxic antibody was neutralized by the intact IVIG and $F(ab')_2$ fragment but not by the Fc fragment [130], implying a antiidiotypic suppression of the cytotoxic IgG.

The ability of IVIG to decrease antibody production may be desirable in patients producing autoantibody, but dangerous in those with infection [153]. Patients with acute otitis were given repeated [22] infusions of IVIG at 3-4 weekly intervals. Such treatment resulted in higher IgG levels if the initial anti-pneumococcal antibodies were low; however, in the presence of high initial levels of antibody, specific anti-pneumococcal antibody levels decreased following this infusion [157]. Others have speculated that high levels of non-specific antibody could lead to a reduction in the survival of specific antibody [158, 159]. There is also suggestive evidence that IVIG may, in some situations, exacerbate infections. Cross et al. described the death of one patient with neutropenia whose infection with yeast accelerated shortly after the infusion of IVIG. It was speculated that the IVIG might have blocked the normal Fc-mediated clearance mechanisms by which the yeast could have been cleared by the host [160]. This possibility was shown to occur in neutropenic mice who were pretreated with high (800 mg/kg) and low (200 mg/kg) IVIG and later challenged with a relatively avirulent strain of *E. coli*. Mice that received the high, but not the low, dose of IVIG had impaired clearance of immune complexes and increased susceptibility to lethal infection [161].

There is additional experimental evidence that IVIG, in conjunction with antimicrobial agents, may, in some circumstances be less efficacious than either alone. The combination of IVIG and ceftriaxone resulted in a higher mortality in infant rats infected with *H. influenzae* type B, than in animals treated with the antibiotic alone [162]. In addition, immunoglobulin therapy alone may have increased the early mortality from this infection. In a similar model that assessed the efficacy of penicillin in conjunction with either albumin or IVIG on group B streptococcal infection, Weisman and Lorenzetti found high dose (2700 mg/kg), but not the low dose (680 mg/kg) delayed bacterial clearance and had no effect on survival [163]. In addition, *in vitro* opsonophagocytosis was decreased by high levels of IVIG. Finally, Kim demonstrated that penicillin therapy of lethal infection with group B streptococcus in this same infant rat model gave a 51 % mortality rate; when immunoglobulin therapy was added to the penicillin treatment, increased mortality occurred following the 2000 mg/kg dose of IVIG but not the 500 mg/kg dose [164]. The mechanisms of these dose-dependent antagonistic interactions between antibiotics and immunoglobulin are not known. Unlike the study of Cross et al. these studies were done with neonatal animals, not in the presence of neutropenia. Phagocytic defects have been described in neonatal cells, however [165].

While the mechanisms of the antagonistic effect of high doses of IVIG are not well defined, the initial observation of this effect was made over 50 years ago. In a series of studies designed to characterize the mouse protection assay that was used to evaluate antipneumococcal serum, Goodner et al. described the phenomenon of fewer animals surviving with progressively larger amounts of serum [166-168]. This "prozone" effect has been described with monoclonal antibodies as well, which suggests the effect is not simply due to the presence of inhibitors in whole serum [169].

Others have found IgG can bind both native C3 and C3b during complement activation by soluble immune complexes and by bacteria [170, 171]. Finally, since immunoglobulin has unique antigenic determinants on it (at the *Gm* and *Inv* loci) antibodies to the immunoglobulin may develop [35, 172]. The physiologic effect of these antibodies has yet to be fully determined, but may conceivably play a role in the anti-idiotype network. In summary, exogenous immunoglobulin has a diverse, potent effect on a wide variety of immune regulatory mechanisms. These interactions may often work to the patient's benefit, but may also result in previously unsuspected adverse effects.

5.9 Adverse Effects (Clinical)

Considerable experience has shown ISG to be one of the safest biological products available. The overall incidence of reactions to ISG is 3-12 % [1]. Janeway found adverse reactions during the treatment of measles to be 1-2 % and mild (see in [173]).

Systemic reactions may occur during or within minutes of administration of ISG. These anaphylactic reactions are quite rare. Late-occuring systemic reactions (hours or days) include arthralgias, pyrexia and diarrhea. Such reactions are not uncommon in immunodeficient patients [36]. Systemic reactions with ISG occur at a rate of approximately 1/500-1 000 injections, and are more common with IVIG. Patients receiving IVIG for hypogammaglobulinemia have a reported incidence of 2.5 % reactions which are usually mild and related to the rate of infusion [30]. The incidence of these reactions decreases after the first 2 months of therapy. Reactions with IVIG often depend on the rate of infusion and the type of preparation. The cause of these reactions with IVIG is not clear but may depend on aggregates, IgA contamination and activated enzymes that initiate the release of inflammatory mediators [36].

Local reactions occur with intramuscular administration of ISG and these are related primarily to the large volumes administered. Local reactions to ISG might be prevented by using small volumes or by pretreatment with analgesics. Systemic reactions may be modified by the use of aspirin, hydrocortisone or antihistamines.

While there are a great number of theoretical reasons derived from experimental work for caution in the use of immunoglobulin (discussed above), there is also well-established clinical experience for such caution. This involves primarily concerns about virus transmission, anaphylactic reactions among patients with IgA deficiency and isolated case reports of unusual occurrences. Even before the advent of IVIG there was sufficient data for one observer to note that gamma globulin administration should no longer be looked upon as inconsequential and that the indications for its use should be sound [35].

Viral Transmission. ISG has had an outstanding record of safety with regard to a lack of transmission of virus to recipients (see [173]). It has been well documented that ISG is free of serum hepatitis, even if the virus is in the original plasma. In England ten children received plasma for prophylaxis against measles. Seven of these children became jaundiced and 3 died. In contrast, ISG prepared from this same plasma was given to 56 children with one child becoming jaundiced [10]. In the United States, 15 volunteers were inoculated subcutaneously with hepatitis-positive plasma. Four of these 15 developed hepatitis. Five received large doses of the ISG and none developed hepatitis [10]. The ability of the Cohn-Oncley fractionation to inactivate virus may in part be due to the high concentration of anti-virus antibody [20]. Non-A, non-B hepatitis (NANB) has been reported in pastes from this procedure: in one, the lyophilization step was omitted, and in 2 others an ion exchange step was added to lower the IgA-content but it lowered the IgG_4-level as well [24].

In contrast, there have been a number of reports of NANB hepatitis following IVIG infusion [174-176]. In one such episode 16/77 patients who received IVIG for immunodeficiency acquired NANB hepatitis with death occuring in 5. Evidence of hepatitis was found in all. Interestingly, no hepatitis was observed following the administration of ISG prepared from the same serum pool [174]. Since none of the products had a recognized virucidal finishing treatment, such as acid treatment, beta-propiolactone or ultraviolet radiation, it is possible that NANB was still viable. Thus ethanol fractionation by itself might not fully inactivate putative virus [177], though it is virucidal for enveloped viruses [178]. With the addition of virucidal procedures to the cold ethanol fractionation step, IVIG could be made safe from NANB hepatitis transmission [178].

Unlike plasma, IVIG has not been known to transmit hepatitis B [179]. There have been no confirmed cases of transmission of HIV virus in IVIG but antibody to HIV has been isolated from 2 patients with primary hypogammaglobulinemia [178]. When HIV was added to plasma and then processed into IVIG, greater than 10^4 pfu/ml of HIV were inactivated during the alcohol fractionation to fractions II and III, and from fractions II and III to fraction II and greater than 10^4 pfu/ml during PEG fractionation of fractions II and III to IVIG [180]. Similar studies by Mitra et al. documented reduction of HIV 10^5- to 10^8-fold in preparing Cohn fraction II, 10^3-10^5-fold through pH 4.0 treatment, and another 10^4-fold through incubation of the purified liquid preparation at 27 °C or 45 °C [181]. Antibody to HIV was detected by ELISA in all 10 lots of a reduced and alkylated IVIG and in 4/8 lots of a pH 4/pepsin IVIG. Eight of these 10 and 3 of these 8 lots were also positive by Western blot analysis. The lots, which were negative for HIV by culture and reverse transcriptase activity, were infused into patients. Comparison of pre- and post-infusion sera demonstrated that antibody to HIV was detectable for up to one month before converting to a negative antibody status [179]. Subsequent reports of seroconversion following the infusion of HIV-antibody positive preparations documented the transient and passive character of this antibody: 6 patients who received IVIG that contained antibody to HIV were seronegative 7-9 months after infusion [182].

Recently one woman who had received hyperimmune Rho(D) immunoglobulin subsequently was found to be infected with HIV. Investigation of samples from the lots of immunoglobulin by the FDA found no HIV antibody or antigen. The plasma used in those lots was screened and found not to contain HIV. Finally examination of records showed that good laboratory practices were maintained throughout production. The woman was found to belong to a group at increased risk of acquiring infection with HIV [183].

Anaphylaxis. Anaphylaxis has been documented to occur following the administration of IVIG to some patients with hypogammaglobulinemia. Indeed patients with antibody deficiency have an increased incidence of adverse reactions to IVIG [9]. In such episodes IgE-antibody to IgA in the infused IVIG was felt to account for these reactions [184]. Low levels of IgA are associated with an increased risk of such anaphylactic reactions [184]. Currently available IVIG products differ markedly in their IgA content [185]. In addition, IgE has been detected in commercial preparations of IVIG [186].

Other clinical problems have been described in case reports: one patient with hypogammaglobulinemia secondary to B cell neoplasm received IVIG prophylaxis. This precipitated cryoglobulinemic nephropathy [187]. The passive transfer of anti-blood-type specific antibody in IVIG may also be associated with a Coombs-positive hemolytic anemia or cause problems in the crossmatching of blood prior to surgery [188]. Immunologically normal patients may get antibody to immunoglobulin that is of a different genotype.

5.10 Conclusions

It is now possible to safely deliver large amounts of immunoglobulin directly into the bloodstream, the need of which was recognized by Cohn over 40 years ago. This has led to the realization that immunoglobulin is itself a potent modulator of the immune system. This observation in turn has resulted in the use of IVIG as a form of therapy for many non-infectious diseases; however, the impact of such treatment on the ability to respond to infectious diseases which often complicate these conditions still must be determined.

Even with the ability to deliver such large doses of immunoglobulin, studies to date have not clearly shown this to expand the indications for its use in infectious diseases beyond those already shown for ISG. In some conditions characterized by functional hypogammaglobulinemia (e. g. HIV infection in young children, chronic lymphocytic leukemia) prophylaxis with standard IVIG may ultimately demonstrate efficacy when the controlled trials are complete.

In certain subpopulations at substantial risk of infection from predictable organisms over a finite period of time, such as the study by Santosham et al. [59] and perhaps in organ transplant patients with respect to CMV, immunoglobulin preparations enriched in antibody to those organisms (hyperimmune) may prove to be useful. The most promising uses appear to be in the prophylaxis of specific infections. These situations usually involve hyperimmune serum and, as shown by studies in neonates, particularly that by Shigeoka et al. [75], the substantial replacement of blood volume. This may be more difficult in the adult.

The use of IVIG to treat established infections with pharmacologic, not replacement doses of immunoglobulin, (with the *possible* exception of antitoxin treatment of septic shock), still has no proven role. This may be in part related to the need for high amounts of *specific* antibody (thus the need for rapid identification of microorganisms) and the need for prompt intervention. Experimental studies in which the exact onset of infection is known, have largely shown that preparations known to be effective in immunotherapy are less efficacious when given 8 hours or more after the onset of infection. A substantial clinical and experimental literature does suggest that passive immunotherapy in conjunction with antimicrobial therapy may provide an enhanced therapeutic benefit; however, this still remains to be shown in a prospective, controlled therapeutic trial.

Finally, it should be noted that most recent studies showing some benefit from passive immunotherapy have not been done with preparations produced as an IVIG (e. g. [56, 71, 77, 79]). Thus despite the substantial progress made in the development of preparations for human use, their firm recommendation for widespread use in infectious disease must still await further well-designed studies.

5.11 References

1. Stiehm, E. R., Ashida, E., Kim, K. S., Winston, D. J., Haas, A. and Gale, R. P., *Ann. Intern. Med.* (1987), **107**, 367-382.
2. Stiehm, E. R., *Pediatr.* (1979), **63**, 301-319.
3. Finlayson, J. A., *In:* Easmon, C. S. F., and Jeljaszewicz, J. (eds.), Medical Microbiology, **vol. 1,** Academic Press, London, (1982), 129-192.
4. Heffron, R., Pneumonia, With Special Reference to *Pneumococcus* Lobar Pneumonia, The Commonwealth Fund, New York, (1939).
5. Roussell, R. H., Collins, M. S., Dobkin, M. B., Louie, R. E., Roby, R. E. and Sweet, B. H., *Amer. J. Med.* (1984), **76, Suppl.**, 40-45.
6. Alexander, H. E., *Amer. J. Dis. Child.* (1943), **66**, 172-187.
7. Alexander, H. E., *Amer. J. Dis. Child.* (1943), **66**, 160-171.
8. Merler, E. and Rosen, F. S., *N. Engl. J. Med.* (1966), **275**, 480-486; 536-542.
9. Janeway, C. A. and Rosen, F. S., *N. Engl. J. Med.* (1966), **275**, 826-831.
10. Stokes, J., Maris, E. P. and Gellis, S. S., *J. Clin. Invest.* (1944), **23**, 531-540.
11. Gross, P., Gitlin, D. and Janeway, C. A., *N. Engl. J. Med.* (1959), **260**, 170-178.
12. Stokes, J. and Neefe, J. R., *J.A.M.A.* (1945), **127**, 531-540.
13. Hammon, W. M., Coriell, L. L., Stokes, J., et al., *J.A.M.A.* (1950), **150**, 739-749; 750-756.
14. Janeway, C. A., Apt, L. and Gitlin, D., *Trans. Ass. Amer. Phycns.* (1953), **66**, 200-202.
15. Gross, P. A. M., Gitlin, D. and Janeway, C. A., *N. Engl. J. Med.* (1959), **260**, 121-125.
16. Hamilton, R. G., *Clin. Chem.* (1987), **33**, 1707-1725.
17. Siber, G. R., Schur, P. H., Weitzman, A. C. and Schifman, G., *N. Engl. J. Med.* (1980), **303**, 178-182.
18. Yount, W. J., Hong, R., Seligmann, M., Good, R. and Kunkel, H. G., *J. Clin. Invest.* (1970), **49**, 1957.
19. Schur, P., Borel, H., Gelfand, E. W., Alper, C. A. and Rosen, F. S., *N. Engl. J. Med.* (1970), **283**, 631.
20. Oxelius, V.-A., *Clin. Exp. Immunol.* (1974), **17**, 19-27.
21. Berger, M., *J. Pediat.* (1987), **110**, 325-328.
22. Schless, A. P. and Harell, G. S., *Amer. J. Med.* (1968), **44**, 325-329.
23. Barandun, S. and Isliker, H., *Vox Sang.* (1986), **51**, 157-160.
24. Hassig, A., *Vox Sang.* (1986), **51**, 10-17.
25. Roifman, C. M., Lederman, H. M., Lavi, S., Stein, L. D., Levison, H. and Gelfand, E. W., *Amer. J. Med.* (1985), **79**, 171-174.
26. Schroeder, D. D. and Dumas, M. L., *Amer. J. Med.* (1984), **76, Suppl.**, 33-39.
27. Janeway, C. A., Merler, E., Rosen, F. S., Salmon, S. and Crain, J. D., *N. Engl. J. Med.* (1968), **278**, 919-923.
28. Passwell, J., Rosen, F. S. and Merler, E., *In:* Alving, B. and Finlayson, J. (eds.), Immunoglobulins: characteristics and uses of intravenous preparations, U.S.Dept. H.H.S., Washington, (1979), 139-142.
29. Ochs, H. D., Fischer, S. H. and Wedgwood, R. J., *J. Clin. Immun.* (1982), **2**, 22S-29S.
30. Cunningham-Rundles, C., Siegal, F. P., Smithwick, E. M., Lion-Boule, A., Cunningham-Rundles, S., O'Malley, J., Barandun, S. and Good, R. A., *Ann. Intern. Med.* (1984), **101**, 435-439.
31. Collins, M. S. and Dorsey, J. H., *J. Infect. Dis.* (1985), **151**, 1171-1173.
32. Schreiber, J. R., Barrus, V. A. and Siber, G. R., *Infect. Immun.* (1985), **47**, 142-148.
33. Ochs, H. D., Buckley, R. H., Pirofsky, B., Fischer, S. H., Roussell, R. R., Anderson, C. J. and Wedgwood, R. J., *Lancet* (1980), **2,** 1158-1159.
34. *Medical Letter* (1982), **24**, 81-82.
35. Ellis, E. F. and Henney, C. S., *J. Allergy* (1969), **43**, 45-54.
36. Cunningham-Rundles, C., Hanson, L. H., Hitzig, W. H., Knapp, W., Lambert, P.-H., Nydegger, U. E., Prince, A. M., Rosen, F. S., Seligmann, M., Soothill, J. E., Thompson, R. A., Torrigiani, G. and Wedgwood, R. J., *Bull. WHO* (1982), **60**, 43-47.

37. Pirofsky, B., *Amer. J. Med.* (1984), **76**, 53-60.
38. Nolte, M. T., Pirofsky, B., Gerritz, G. A. and Golding, B., *Clin. Exp. Immunol.* (1979), **36**, 237-243.
39. Berkman, S. A., Lee, M. L. and Gale, R. P., *Semin. Hemat.* (1988), **25**, 140-158.
40. Buckley, R. H., *J. Clin. Immunol.* (1982), **2**, 15S-21S.
41. Ochs, H. D., Fischer, S. H. and Wedgwood, R. J., *J. Clin. Immunol.* (1982), **2**, 22S-30S.
42. Stiehm, E. R., Vaerman, J.-P. and Fudenberg, H. H., *Blood* (1966), **28**, 918-937.
43. Gonzalez, E. B., Guernsey, B. G., Ingrim, N. B., Ichikawa, Y. and Daniels, J. C., *Arch. Intern. Med.* (1985), **145**, 945-946.
44. Christensen, K. K., Christensen, P., Bucher, H. U., Duc, G., Kind, C. H., Mieth, D., Buller, B. and Seger, R. A., *Eur. J. Pediatr.* (1984), **143**, 123-127.
45. Krugman, S., *N. Engl. J. Med.* (1963), **269**, 195-201.
46. Grossman, E. B., Stewart, S. G. and Stokes, J., *J.A.M.A.* (1945), **129**, 991-994.
47. Medical Research Council Working-party, *Lancet* (1969), **1**, 163-168.
48. Leen, C. L. S., Yap, P. L. and McClelland, D. B. L., *Vox Sang.* (1986), **51**, 278-286.
49. Editorial, *Lancet* (1983), **1**, 105-106.
50. Chirico, G., Rondini, G., Plebani, A., Chiara, A., Massa, M. and Ugazi, A. G., *J. Pediatr.* (1987), **110**, 437-442.
51. Amer, J., Ott, E., Ibbott, F. A., O'Brien, D. and Kempe, C. H., *Pediatr.* (1963), **32**, 4-9.
52. Hertler, A. A. and Ross, S. C., *J. Clin. Lab. Immunol.* (1986), **21**, 177-181.
53. Baron, S., Barnet, E. V., Goldsmith, R. S., Silbergeld, S., Ehrmantraut, W. R., Boyland, J. E. and Burch, B. L., *Amer. J. Hyg.* (1964), **79**, 186-195.
54. Kefalides, N. A., Arana, J. A., Bazan, A., Bocanegra, M., Stastny, P., Velarde, N. and Rosenthal, S. M., *N. Engl. J. Med.* (1962), **267**, 317-324.
55. Stone, H. H., Graber, C. D., Martin, J. D. and Kolb, L., *Surgery* (1965), **58**, 810-814.
56. Jones, R. J., Roe, E. A. and Gupta, J. L., *Lancet* (1980), **2**, 1263-1265.
57. Wasserman, R. L., *Pediatr. Infect. Dis.* (1986), **5**, 620-621.
58. Steen, J. A., *Arch. Pediatr.* (1960), **77**, 291-294.
59. Santosham, M., Reid, R., Ambrusino, D. M., Wolff, M. C., Almeido-Hill, J., Priehs, C., Aspery, K. M., Garrett, S., Croll, L., Foster, S., Burge, G., Page, P., Zacher, B., Moxon, R. and Siber, G. R., *N. Engl. J. Med.* (1987), **317**, 923-929.
60. Conway, S. P., Gillies, D. R. N. and Docherty, A., *Arch. Dis. Child.* (1987), **62**, 1252-1256.
61. Sidiropoulos, D., Herrmann, U., Morell, A., von Muralt, G. and Barandun, S., *J. Pediatr.* (1986), **109**, 505-508.
62. Haque, K. N., Zaidi, M. H., Haque, S. K., Bahakim, H., El-Hazmi, M. and El-Swailam, M., *Pediatr. Infect. Dis.* (1986), **5**, 622-625.
63. Haque, K. N., Zaidi, M. H. and Bahakim, H., *Amer. J. Dis. Child.* (1988), **142**, 1293-1296.
64. Stabile, A., Miceli Sopo, S., Romanelli, V., Pastore, M. and Pesaresis, M. A., *Arch. Dis. Child.* (1988), **63**, 441-443.
65. Rosenthal, S. M., Millican, R. C. and Rust, J., *Proc. Soc. Exp. Biol. Med.* (1957), **94**, 214-217.
66. Fisher, M. W., *Antibiot. Chemother.* (1957), **7**, 315-321.
67. Fisher, M. W. and Manning, M. C., *Antibiot. Chemother.* (1958), **81**, 29-31.
68. Waisbren, B. A., *Antibiot. Chemother.* (1957), **7**, 322-333.
69. Waisbren, B. A. and Lepley, D., *Arch. Intern. Med.* (1962), **109**, 712-716.
70. Bodey, G. P., Nies, B. A., Mohberg, N. R. and Freireich, E. J., *J.A.M.A.* (1964), **190**, 1099-1102.
71. Finkel, K. C. and Haworth, J. C., *Pediatr.* (1960), **25**, 798-806.
72. Feingold, D. S. and Oski, F., *Arch. Intern. Med.* (1965), **126**, 226-228.
73. Millican, R. C. and Rust, J. D., *J. Infect. Dis.* (1960), **107**, 389-394.
74. Forman, M. L. and Stiehm, R., *N. Engl. J. Med.* (1969), **281**, 926-931.
75. Shigeoka, A. S., Hall, R. T. and Hill, H. R., *Lancet* (1978), **1**, 636-638.
76. Ziegler, E. J., McCutchan, J. A., Fierer, J., Glauser, M. P., Sadoff, J. C., Douglas, H. and Braude, A. I., *New Engl. J. Med.* (1982), **307**, 1225-1230.
77. Baumgartner, J.-D., Glauser, M. P., McCutchan, J. A., Ziegler, E. J., van Melle, G., Klauber, M. R., Vogt, M., Muehlen, E., Luethy, R., Chiolero, R. and Geroulanos, S., *Lancet* (1985), **2**, 59-63.

78. Calandra, T., Schellekens, J., Verhoef, J. and Glauser, M. P., *In:* Program and Abstracts for the 4th International Symposium on Infections in the Immunocompromised Host. Ronneby Brunn, Sweden (1986), Abstract **No. 128.**
79. Lachman, E., Pitsoe, S.B. and Gaffin, S. L., *Lancet* (1984), **1**, 981-983.
80. Thomson, M. A., *J. S. Afr. Vet. Ass.* (1983), **54**, 279-281.
81. Exley, A. R., Buurman, W., Hanson, G., Owen, R., Riddell, A. and Cohen, J., Abstr. **324** of 29th Interscience Conference on Antimicrobial Agents and Chemotherapy, Houston, TX, (1989).
82. Snydman, D. R., Werner, B. G., Heinze-Lacey, B., Berardi, V. P., Tilney, N. L., Kirkman, R. L., Milford, E. L., Cho, S. L., Bush, H. L., Levey, A. S., Strom, T. B., Carpenter, C. B., Levey, R. H., Harmon, W. E., Zimmerman, C. E., Shapiro, M. E., Steinman, T., LoGerfo, F., Idelson, B., Schroter, G. P. J., Levin, M. J., McIver, J., Leszczynski, J. and Grady, G. F., *N. Engl. J. Med.* (1987), **317**, 1049-1054.
83. Condie, R. M. and O'Reilly, R. J., *Amer. J. Med.* (1984), **76, Suppl.**, 134-141.
84. Winston, D. J., Ho, W. G., Lin, C.-H., Budinger, M. D., Champlin, R. E. and Gale, R. P., *Amer. J. Med.* (1984), **76, Suppl.**, 128-133.
85. Hagenbeek, A., Brummelhuis, H. G. J., Donkers, A., Dumas, A. M., ten Haaft, A., Schaapl, B. J. P., Sizoo, W. and Lowenberg, B., *J. Infect. Dis.* (1987), **155**, 897-902.
86. Bowden, R. A., Sayers, M., Flournoy, N., Newton, B., Banaji, M., Thomas, E. D. and Meyers, J. D., *N. Engl. J. Med.* (1986), **314**, 1006-1010.
87. Reed, E. C., Bowden, R. A., Dandliker, P. S., Gleaves, C. A. and Meyers, J. D., *J. Infect. Dis.* (1987), 641-644.
88. Emanuel, E., Cunningham, I., Jules-Elysee, K., Brochstein, J. A., Kernan, N. A., Laver, J., Stover, D., White, D. A., Fels, A., Polsky, B., Castro-Malaspina, H., Peppard, J. R., Bartus, P., Hammerling, U. and O'Reilly, R. J., *Ann. Intern. Med.* (1988), **109**, 777-782.
89. Reed, E. C., Bowden, R. A., Dandliker, P. S., Lilleby, K. E. and Meyers, J. D., *Ann. Intern. Med.* (1988), **109**, 783-788.
90. Kasiske, B. L., Heim-Duthoy, K. L., Tortorice, K. L., Ney, A. L., Odland, M. D. and Rao, K. V., *Arch. Intern. Med.* (1989), **149**, 2733-2736.
91. Erlendsson, K., Swartz, T. and Dwyer, J. M., *N. Engl. J. Med.* (1985), **312**, 351-353.
92. Mease, P. J., Ochs, H. D. and Wedgwood, R. J., *N. Engl. J. Med.* (1981), **304**, 1278-1281.
93. Crennan, J. M., van Scoy, R. E., McKenna, C. H. and Smith, T. F., *Amer. J. Med.* (1986), **81**, 35-42.
94. Erlich, K. S. and Mills, J., *Rev. Infect. Dis.* (1986), **8**, S439-S445.
95. Ho, W. G., Winston, D. J., Bartoni, K., Champlin, R. R. and Gale, R. P., Abstr. **456**, Interscience Confer. Infect. Dis. Chemother, Las Vegas, Nevada, (1983).
96. Cooperative Group for the Study of Immunoglobulin in Chronic Lymphocytic Leukemia, *N. Engl. J. Med.* (1988), **319**, 902-907.
97. Ochs, H. D., *Pediatr. Infect. Dis.* (1987), **6**, 509-511.
98. Wood, C. C., McNamara, J. G., Schwarz, D. E., Merrill, W. W. and Shapiro, E. D., *Pediatr. Infect. Dis.* (1987), **6**, 565-566.
99. Silverman, B. A. and Rubinstein, A., *Amer. J. Med.* (1985), **78**, 728-736.
100. Sidiropoulos, D., Boehme, U., von Muralt, G., Morell, A. and Barandun, S., *Pediatr. Infect. Dis.* (1986), **5**, S193-S194.
101. Sumer, T., Abumelha, A., Al-Mulhim, I. and Al-Fadil, M., *Eur. J. Pediatr.* (1989), **148**, 401-402.
102. Winnie, G. B., Cowan, R. G. and Wade, N. A., *J. Pediatr.* (1989), **114**, 309-314.
103. Ambrosino, D., Schreiber, J. R., Daum, R. S. and Siber, G. R., *Infet. Immun.* (1983), **39**, 709-714.
104. Harper, T. E., Christensen, R. D. and Rothstein, G., *Ped. Res.* (1987), **22**, 455-460.
105. Cryz, S. J., Cross, A. S., Furer, E., Chariatte, N., Sadoff, J. C. and Germanier, R., *J. Lab. Clin. Med.* (1986), **108**, 182-189.
106. Holder, I. A. and Naglich, J. G., *Amer. J. Med.* (1984), **76**, 161-167.
107. Pennington, J. E. and Small, G. J., *J. Infect. Dis.* (1987), **155**, 973-978.
108. Hemming, V. G., London, W. T., Fischer, G. W., Curfman, B. L., Baron, P. A., Gloser, H., Bachmayer, H. and Wilson, S. R., *J. Infect. Dis.* (1987), **156**, 655-658.
109. Ashkenazi, S., Cleary, T. G., Lopez, E. and Pickering, L. K., *J. Pediatr.* (1988), **113**, 1008-1014.

110. Kim, K. S., Dunn, K., McGeary, S. A. and Stiehm, E. R., *Pediatr. Res.* (1984), **18**, 1329-1331.
111. Eibl, M. M., Wolf, I. H. M., Furnkranz, H. and Rosenkranz, A., *N. Engl. J. Med.* (1988), **319**, 1-7.
112. Mietens, C., Keinhorst, H., Hilpert, H., Gerber, H., Amster, H. and Pahud, J. J., *Eur. J. Pediatr.* (1979), **132**, 239-252.
113. Tacket, C. O., Losonsky, G., Link, H., Hoang, Y., Guesry, P., Hilpert, H. and Levine, M. M., *N. Engl. J. Med.* (1988), **318**, 1240-1243.
114. Rubin, R. R., Fischman, A. J., Callahan, R. J., Khaw, B.-A., Keech, F., Ahmad, M., Wilkinson, R. and Strauss, H. W., *N. Engl. J. Med.* (1989), **321**, 935-940.
115. Barandun, S., Imbach, P., Morrell, A., Wagner, H. P., *In:* Nydegger, U. E. (ed.), Immunohemotherapy. A guide to immunoglobulin prophylaxis and therapy, Academic Press, New York, (1981), 275-282.
116. Imbach, P., Wagner, H. P., Berchtold, W., Gaedicke, G., Hirt, A., Joller, P., Mueller-Eckhardt, C., Muller, B., Rossi, E. and Barandun, S., *Lancet* (1985), **2**, 464-468.
117. Fehr, J., Hoffmann, V. and Kappeler, U., *N. Engl. J. Med.* (1982), **306**, 1254-1258.
118. Rosthoj, S., Steffensen, G. K. and Guld, T. K., *Acta Paediatr. Scand.* (1987), **76**, 631-635.
119. Leickly, F. E. and Buckley, R. H., *Amer. J. Med.* (1987), **82**, 159-162.
120. Richmond, G. W., Ray, I. and Korenblitt, A., *J. Pediatr.* (1987), **110**, 917-919.
121. Hilgartner, M. W. and Bussel, J., *Amer. J. Med.* (1987), **83**, 35-39.
122. Becker, T., Panzer, S., Maas, D., Kiefel, V., Sprenger, R., Kirschbaum, M. and Mueller-Eckhardt, I. C., *Brit. J. Haemat.* (1985), **61**, 149-155.
123. Dammacco, E., Iodice, G. and Campobasso, N., *Brit. J. Haemat.* (1986), **62**, 125-135.
124. Newland, A. C., Treleaven, J. G., Minchinton, R. M., Waters, A. H., *Lancet* (1983), **1**, 84-87.
125. Bussel, J. B., Kimberly, R. P., Inman, R. D., Schulman, I., Cunningham-Rundles, C., Cheung, N., Smithwick, E. M., O'Malley, J., Barandun, S. and Hilgartner, M. W., *Blood* (1983), **62**, 480-486.
126. Duran-Suarez, J.R., Martin, A., Botella, M. C., de la Torre, S., Bailen, A. and Maldonado, J., *Haematologica* (1983), **68**, 564-566.
127. Schiffer, C. A., Hogge, D. E., Aisner, J., Dutcher, J. P., Lee, E. J. and Pappenberg, D., *Blood* (1984), **64**, 937-940.
128. Chirico, G., Duse, M., Ugazio, A. G. and Rondini, G., *J. Pediatr.* (1983), **103**, 654-655.
129. Besa, E. C., McNab, M. W., Solan, A. J., Lapes, M. J. and Marfatia, U., *Amer. J. Hematol.* (1985), **18**, 373-379.
130. McGuire, W. A., Yang, H. H., Bruno, E., Brandt, J., Briddell, R., Coates, T. D. and Hoffman, R., *N. Engl. J. Med.* (1987), **317**, 1004-1008.
131. De La Camara, C., Arrieta, R., Gonzales, A., Iglesias, E. and Omenaca, F., *N. Engl. J. Med.* (1988), **318**, 519-520.
132. Nilsson, I. M., Berntorp, E. and Zettervall, O., *N. Engl. J. Med.* (1988), **318**, 947-950.
133. Bohm, R., Hofstaetter, C. and Briel, R. C., *Blut* (1984), **48**, 469-470.
134. Newburger, J. W., Takahashe, M., Burns, J. C., Beiser, A. S., Chung, K. J., Duffy, C. E., Glode, M. P., Mason, W. H., Reddy, V., Sanders, S. P., Shulman, S. T., Wiggins, J. W., Hicks, R. V., Fulton, D. R., Lewis, A. B., Leung, D. Y. M., Colton, T., Tosen, F. S. and Melish, M. E., *N. Engl. J. Med.* (1986), **315**, 341-347.
135. Nagashima, M., Matsushima, M., Matsuoka, H., Ogawa, A. and Okumara, N., *J. Pediatr.* (1987), **110**, 710-712.
136. Leung, D. Y. M., Burns, J. C., Newburger, J. W. and Geha, R. S., *J. Clin. Invest.* (1987), **79**, 468-472.
137. Breedveld, F. C., Brand, A. and van Aken, W. G., *J. Rheumat.* (1985), **12**, 700-702.
138. Arsura, E. L., Bick, A. S., Brunner, N. G., Namba, T. and Grob, D., *Arch. Intern. Med.* (1986), **146**, 1365-1368.
139. Kawada, K. and Terasaki, P. I., *Exp. Hematol.* (1987), **15**, 133-136.
140. Schuller, E. and Govaerts, A., *Europ. Neurol.* (1983), **22**, 205-212.
141. Combe, B., Cosso, B., Clot, J., Bonneau, M. and Sany, J., *Amer. J. Med.* (1985), **78**, 920-992.
142. Salama, A., Mueller-Eckhardt, C. and Kiefel, V., *Lancet* (1983), **2**, 193-195.
143. Kimberly, R. P., Salmon, J. E., Bussel, J., Crow, M. K. and Hilgartner, M. W., *J. Immunol.* (1984), **132**, 745-750.

144. Budde, U., Auch, D., Niese, D., Schafer, G., Reske, S. N. and Schmidt, R. E., *Scand. J. Haemat.* (1986), **37**, 125-129.
145. Etzioni, A., Pollack, S. and Benderly, A., *N. Engl. J. Med.* (1988), **318**, 994.
146. Sandilands, G. P., Atrah, H. I., Templeton, G., Cocker, J. E., Lucie, N, Crawford, R. J. and MacSween, R. N. M., *J. Clin. Lab. Immunol.* (1987), **23**, 109-115.
147. Kurtzman, G., Frickhofen, N., Kimball, J., Jenkins, D. W., Nienhuis, A. W. and Young, N. S., *N. Engl. J. Med.*
148. Engelhard, D., Waner, J. L., Kapoor, N. and Good, R. A., *J. Pediatr.* (1986), **108**, 77-81.
149. Besa, E. C., *Amer. J. Med.* (1984), **76**, 209-218.
150. Cook, L., Howard, J. F., Jr. and Folds, J. D., *J. Clin. Immunol.* (1988), **8**, 23-31.
151. Barbano, G., Saleh, M. N., Mori, P. G., LoBuglio, A. F. and Shaw, D. R., *Blood* (1989), **73**, 662-665.
152. Jungi, T. W. and Barandun, S., *Vox Sang.* (1985), **49**, 9-19.
153. Stohl, W., *Clin. Exp. Immunol.* (1985), **62**, 200-207.
154. Hashimoto, F., Sakiyama, Y. and Matsumoto, S., *Clin. Exp. Immunol.* (1986), **65**, 409-415.
155. Hodes, H. H., *Pediatr.* (1963), **32**, 1-3.
156. White, W. B., Desbonnet, C. R. and Ballow, M., *Amer. J. Med.* (1987), **83**, 431-444.
157. Prellner, W. B., Christensen, P., Kalm, O. and Offenbartl, K., *Acta Path. Microbiol. Immunol. Scand. Sect. C* (1986), **94**, 207-211.
158. Christensen, K. K. and Christensen, P., *Pediatr. Infect. Dis.* (1986), **5**, S189-S192.
159. Kelton, J. G., Carter, C. J., Rodger, C., Bebenek, G., Gauldie, J., Sheridan, D., Kassam, Y. B., Kean, W. E., Buchanan, W. W., Rooney, P. J., Bianchi, F. and Denburg, J., *Blood* (1984), **63**, 1434-1438.
160. Cross, A. S., Alving, B. M., Sadoff, J. C., Baldwin, P., Terebelo, H. and Tang, D., *Lancet* (1984), **1**, 912.
161. Cross, A. S., Siegel, G., Byrne, W. R., Trautmann, . and Finbloom, D. S., *Clin. Exp. Immunol.* (1989), **76**, 159-164.
162. Schreiber, J., Basker, C., Priehs, C. and Siber, G., *Pediatr. Res.* (1987), **21**, 334A.
163. Weisman, L. E. and Lorenzetti, P. M., *J. Pediatr.* (1989), **115**, 445-450.
164. Kim, K. S., *J. Allergy Clin. Immunol.* (1989), **84**, 579-587.
165. Forman, M. L. and Stiehm, E. R., *N. Engl. J. Med.* (1969), **281**, 926-931.
166. Goodner, K. and Horsfall, F. L., *J. Exp. Med.* (1935), **62**, 359-374.
167. Goodner, K. and Miller, D. K., *J. Exp. Med.* (1935), **62**, 375-391.
168. Goodner, K. and Miller, D. K., *J. Exp. Med.* (1935), **62**, 393-407.
169. Cross, A. S., Zollinger, W., Mandrell, R., Gemski, P. and Sadoff, J., *J. Infect. Dis.* (1983), **147**, 68-76.
170. Berger, M., Rosencranz, P. and Brown, C. Y., *Clin. Immunol. Immunopath.* (1985), **34**, 227-236.
171. Kulics, J., Rajnavolgyi, E., Fust, G. and Gergely, J., *Molecul. Immunol.* (1983), **20**, 805-810.
172. Williams, R. C., Mellbye, O. J. and Kronvall, G., *Infect. Immun.* (1972), **6**, 316-323.
173. Bjorkander, J., Cunningham-Rundles, C., Lundin, P., Olsson, R., Soderstrom, R. and Hanson, L. A., *Amer. J. Med.* (1988), **84**, 107-111.
175. Lane, R. S., *Lancet* (1983), **2**, 974-975.
176. Ochs, H. D., Fischer, S. H., Virant, F. S., Lee, M. L., Kingdom, H. S. and Wedgwood, R. J., *Lancet* (1985), **1**, 404-405.
177. Leen, C. L. S., Yap, P. L., Neill, G., McClelland, D. B. L. and Westwood, A., *Vox Sang.* (1986), **50**, 26-32.
178. Cuthbertson, B., Perry, R. J., Foster, P. R., Reid, K. G., Crawford, R. J. and Yap, P. L., *J. Infect.* (1987), **15**, 125-133.
179. Wood, C. C., Williams, A. E., McNamara, J. G., Annunziata, J. A., Feorino, P. M. and Conway, C. O., *Ann. Intern. Med.* (1986), **105**, 536-538.
180. Hamamoto, Y., Harada, S., Yamamoto, N., Uemura, Y., Goto, T. and Suyama, T., *Vox Sang.* (1987), **53**, 65-69.
181. Mitra, G., Wong, M. E., Mozen, M. M., McDougal, J. S. and Levy, J. A., *Transfusion* (1986), **26**, 394-397.
182. Abacioglu, H. and Okuyan, M., *J. Infect. Dis.* (1989), **160**,.

183. Anon., *Morb. Mortal. Weekly Rpt.* (1987), **36**, 728-729.
184. Burks, A. W., Sampson, H. A. and Buckley, R. H., *New Engl. J. Med.* (1985), **314**, 560-564.
185. Apfelzweig, R., Piskiewicz, D. and Hooper, J. A., *J. Clin. Immunol.* (1987), **7**, 46-50.
186. Paganelli, R., Quinti, I., D'Offizi, G. P., Papetti, C., Cabello, A. and Aiuti, F., *Vox Sang.* (1986), **51**, 87-91.
187. Barton, J. C., Herrera, G. A., Galla, J. H., Bertoli, L. F., Work, J. and Koopman, W. J., *Amer. J. Med.* (1987), **82**, 624-629.
188. Brox, A. G., Cournoyer, D., Sternbach, M. and Spurll, G., *Amer. J. Med.* (1987), **82**, 633-635.

6. Treatment of Infectious Diseases with Monoclonal Antibodies

James W. Larrick

6.1 Introduction

When a vertebrate is vaccinated with a foreign antigen, it produces a mixture of antibodies that can bind to the antigen. Each antibody binds to a different epitope on the immunogen and is made by an individual clone of B lymphocytes. Industrial quantities of a single (i. e., monoclonal) antibody recognizing a specific epitope can be made by fusing a B lymphocyte producing the antibody of interest with an immortal tumor cell line to give hybridomas.

Since the original report in 1975 [1], the generation of rodent monoclonal antibodies (mabs) has become a routine endeavor. The potential of mabs, particularly human mabs (humabs) for therapeutic purposes, was recognized by the first investigators of this technology. However, fifteen years later only limited therapeutic applications have been made due at least in some part to the difficulty of generating humabs. Recent advances with improved fusion partners, *in vitro* immunization and, as discussed below, recombinant DNA approaches may alleviate these shortcomings.

At the present time only two mabs, OKT3 - a murine mab directed against a T-lymphocyte antigen (CD3), and an anti-digoxin mab [2] are licensed drugs. Despite this modest beginning a large number of anti-infectious disease mabs are in clinical development and the technology represents a significant pharmacological advance.

As therapeutic agents, antibodies are not without their problems (see Tab. 6-1). Among these are their protein composition; they are immunogenic [3]; they must be given parenterally; and they are relatively expensive to produce. However, since many therapeutic antibodies are aimed at the treatment of acute life-threatening disease, cost may be of less importance.

Tab. 6-1 Limitations of antibodies as pharmacological agents.

Protein composition
Immunogenicity
Tissue distribution, (Mr)
Parenteral administration
Cost

6.2 Human Monoclonal Antibodies

Antibodies are composed of disulfide-linked heavy and light chains each comprised of variable and constant domains. The most immunogenic portion of antibodies will be the species conserved constant regions.

Humabs will minimize the problems encountered when administering a foreign animal monoclonal antibody (e. g., anaphylaxis, clinical manifestations of immune complex formation, and reduction of efficacy by anti-antibodies). In well over half of the patients treated to date with murine monoclonal antibodies, the human anti-mouse antibody (HAMA) response has limited their usefulness [4]. Only a fraction of the antimouse immune response is directed to the variable region (idiotype) of the rodent immunoglobulins. This suggests that humabs will be more effective therapeutic molecules than their rodent counterparts. Preliminary pharmacokinetic studies with humabs demonstrate the superiority of these molecules over foreign mouse mabs [5].

There are a limited number of clinical settings (see Tab. 6-2) for which passively administered human antisera against specific antigens are currently in use. Humabs that recognize many of these antigens have been produced and will probably augment or replace pooled antisera in the near future.

Tab. 6-2 Clinical settings in which passively administered human antisera against specific target antigens are currently in use/testing.

Red cell antigens	Rh (hemolytic disease of the newborn)
White cell antigens	Antilymphocyte/thymocyte globulin
Viral antigens	Hepatitis A and B
	Rabies,
	Cytomegalovirus,
	Herpes simplex
	Varicella zoster
Bacterial antigens	Tetanus,
	Haemophilus influenzae,
	Endotoxins,
	Pneumococcus
Antisnake venom	
Elimination of circulating drugs (overdoses)	
Fertility control (e. g., anti-beta human chorionic gonadotropin)	

Concerns, which include the possible contamination of pooled globulins by infectious agents (e. g. human immunodeficiency virus, HIV), various hepatitis viruses and cytomegalovirus, and the diminished availability of serum donors, as well as the relative ease of reproducible humab manufacture, will accelerate this trend.

Humabs are more likely to have species-specific carbohydrates which may be important in a number of effector functions, such as Fc receptor-mediated antibody-dependent cellular cytotoxicity, complement activation, and phagocytosis [6]. Serum half-life and effector functions of immunoglobulin subclasses are very important for designing the optimal anti-infectious disease monoclonal antibody therapeutic.

Technology for the generation of therapeutic humabs has lagged behind that developed for rodent mabs. In recent years the development of improved fusion partners with a higher fusion efficiency, greater stability and higher levels of antibody production, as well as advances in the molecular biology of immunoglobulins has reduced the effort to obtain humabs directly or to "humanize" (see below) rodent monoclonals. Another alternative not widely explored until recently is the use of primate monoclonals. Sequences of these proteins are virtually identical to their human counterparts.

In recent years, reproducible reliable techniques for the *in vitro* immunization of human B cells [7] have been developed. These methods combined with the development of immunodeficient mice [8] for the reconstitution of the human immune system *ex vivo* may enhance our capacity to generate humabs of defined specificity. Several recent reviews summarize progress in the generation of humabs [9-11].

6.3 Second Generation Monoclonal Antibodies

6.3.1 Genetically Engineered Monoclonal Antibodies

Several laboratories have used recombinant DNA technology to construct chimaeric rodent-human monoclonal antibodies by attaching human constant regions to the rodent variable regions [12, 13], for review see [14]. Because the antibody combining site is localized within the variable regions these molecules maintain their combining affinity for the antigen and acquire the function of the substituted constant regions [15, 16].

In a more sophisticated approach human antibodies with genetically engineered variable regions have been constructed from rodent monoclonals by splicing the rodent hypervariable, complementarity determining regions (CDRs) onto human conserved framework sequences. Short of deriving a human monoclonal antibody from a human B cell this is about as "humanized" as a rodent monoclonal can become. In one case these 'composite' monoclonals had a combining affinity equal to the parent murine antibody [17]; in the other the affinity was less [18]. The rat anti-CAMPATH-1 monoclonal [19] has been the most successful therapeutic mab humanized to date. This mab recognizes an antigen expressed on virtually all human lymphocytes and monocytes, but is absent from the hematopoietic stem cells. Depletion of cells bearing this antigen appears to be an important therapeutic approach for control of graft-versus-host disease in bone marrow transplantation, prevention of bone marrow and other organ rejection episodes and for treatment of various lymphoid malignancies [20]. The six hypervariable regions from the heavy and light-chain variable region domains of the rat antibody grafted onto the framework regions of a human IgG_1 antibody yielded a 'reshaped' human monoclonal antibody with effector functions equal to (complement fixation) or better (cell-mediated lysis of human lymphocytes) than the parent CAMPATH-1 monoclonal. In the initial clinical trials this pioneer reshaped antibody yielded positive results [21].

It should be noted that even fully humanized mabs may be immunogenic. Although limited studies have demonstrated that the chimaeric mouse-human antibody 17-1A was less immunogenic in humans than the parent mouse monoclonal [25], more studies will be required to determine how much of a problem the human anti-idiotype response will be. In principle, the idiotype of a reshaped recombinant monoclonal could be changed by altering the CDRs or framework regions. However, grafting the CDRs into several cassettes might focus the immune response onto the combining site. This might be one method to potentiate development of effective anti-idiotype vaccines.

6.3.2 Rapid Direct Cloning of Antibody Variable Regions

A major problem with the generation of human monoclonal antibodies is the immortalization of antigen-specific human B cells. Typically this is performed with the aid of Epstein-Barr virus transformation followed by subcloning, testing for antigen binding and hybridizing the B lymphoblasts to a suitable fusion partner such as GLI-H7. [Heteromyeloma fusion partner GLI-H7 is available from the author.] This general approach is effective and widely used, however it is time consuming and erratic immortalization occurs. For this reason, we recently have devised methods to directly obtain the variable regions from a small number of interesting human B cells and the technology is at hand to replace cell fusion as a means of generating monoclonal antibodies.

Fig. 6-1 shows the application of the gene amplification technology (polymerase chain reaction) to immunoengineering. A mixture of oligomer primers in the 5' leader sequences combined with 3' constant region primers permits the amplification of any human immunoglobulin variable region from very small numbers of cells [22-24]. These fragments can be directly sequenced and/or ligated into expression vectors. The method has been used to obtain variable regions of both heavy and light chains from single human B lymphocytes. Thus the variable region genes of B cells can be obtained from *in vitro* antigen expanded cultures or from peripheral blood on the appropriate day post immunization. Fig. 6-1 presents a flow diagram of the steps required to produce recombinant antibodies without cell fusion.

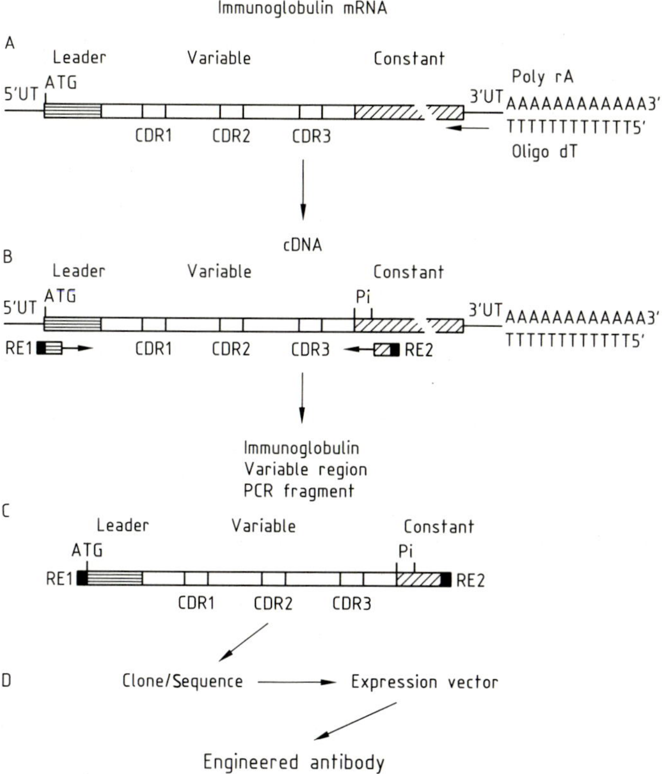

Fig. 6-1 Immunoengineering of antibodies using the polymerase chain reaction. Primers corresponding to conserved regions of the immunoglobulin cDNA are used to amplify the variable regions. These regions can be cloned, sequenced and directly ligated into a vector for expression of an engineered antibody.

6.4 Antibodies to Infectious Diseases

Animal and human antisera have been used for passive immunotherapy of infectious diseases since the turn of the century. Tab. 6-2 lists the clinical settings for which antisera are currently in use. Human monoclonal antibodies will eventually replace all of these antisera. Other uses of immunoglobulins have been reviewed [26].

6.4.1 Bacterial Targets

Various bacterial antigens are recognized by humabs (see Tab. 6-3). Tetanus neutralizing humabs have been frequently generated because of the ease of obtaining immune B cells from vaccinated persons [27-31]. Because tetanus immunization in the United States is universal and most individuals have relatively high titers, it is unlikely that any of these monoclonals will be scaled up and used in the USA. The same is true of anti-diphtheria monoclonal antibodies [32]. In other countries, vaccination against tetanus and diphtheria is not widespread and administration of immune human or animal sera is still practiced. Recent concern about HIV contaminated serum has stimulated efforts to generate humabs against tetanus for use in Asia, South America, and southern Europe.

Tab. 6-3 Human monoclonal antibodies: Bacterial targets.

Tetanus toxoid
Diphtheria toxoid
Gram-negative endotoxins
Pseudomonas aeruginosa
Lipopolysaccharide
Exotoxin A
Haemophilus influenzae
Mycobacterium leprae
Neisseria meningitides [86]
Pneumococcus [87, 88]

Gram-negative bacterial infections account for 1-2 % of hospital admissions and up to 100 000 deaths each year in the USA. Despite currently available therapies including antibiotics and various support measures mortality rates remain as high as 50-70 %. Much interest has been generated by the idea that lipopolysaccharide, the lethal component of Gram-negative bacteria, might have antigenic determinants that are shared by many bacterial species. Lipopolysaccharides have a tripartite structure. Each LPS containing bacterial species is distinguished by its so-called "O" or somatic antigens which are the repeating oligosaccharide subunits. Connected to this region is the LPS "core" composed of a group of sugars conserved across bacterial species and the biologically most toxic portion of the LPS molecule, lipid A. While there are minor differences in the fatty acid chains attached to the diglucosamine framework of lipid A, it is thought that the lipid A portion of LPS is highly conserved across bacterial species [33]. A concept has been the suggestion that lipopolysaccharides share common immunogenic determinants in the core-lipid A portion of the molecules.

Bacteria containing the full complement of lipid A, core carbohydrate and O antigens have a smooth phenotype. Those with mutations of enzymes catalyzing the addition of core sugars are called rough (R) mutants. Tate et al. [34] found that antisera to the core-LPS gave significant protection against endotoxin from a smooth strain of *E. coli* and Chedid et al. [35] reported that hyperimmune serum against rough *Salmonella typhimurium* protected mice against lethal infection with smooth cultures of *Klebsiella pneumoniae.* Braude et al. (review, [36]) and Johns et al. [37] laid the groundwork for the first clinical studies using cross-reactive anti-endotoxin antisera [38]. Recent clinical [39, 40], animal [41] and binding [42] studies have brought the validity of the "core concept" into question as discussed below. Structural data support the existence of cross-reactive determinants across Gram-negative bacterial species. What is lacking is agreement on whether antibodies recognizing these epitopes can block the toxic effects of endotoxin and/or the bacteria that release it.

In the major clinical trial to test the "core concept" antisera were obtained from firemen vaccinated with a rough mutant *E. coli* strain called J5 that lacks the outer carbohydrate. This antiserum gave significant protection to patients with Gram-negative sepsis [43]. Several points are worth emphasizing about this study. Preimmune titers were 1:6 and post-immune titers were 1:32. A dilution of a unit of this J5 antiserum into the average plasma volume would be a dilution of less than 1:50. Thus the final serum titer in treated patients was less than the average pre-immune titer in the vaccinated donors. This study used sera. No attempt was made to demonstrate that antibodies to endotoxin were the active principle in these sera. Acute phase sera or "tolerant" sera contain a number of ill-defined mediators and substances that can apparently neutralize endotoxin. Finally, the J5 antisera were never shown to bind to the organisms causing the severe infections in this study. Several investigators have shown that endotoxin immunization can cause a polyclonal type-specific response. Because many pathogenic strains carry cross-reactive antigens with endogenous flora, augmentation of type-specific titers by vaccination might account for the protective effect of the J5 antisera. Thus for a number of reasons the so-called core concept is questionable.

Several laboratories have demonstrated production of mouse monoclonal antibodies reactive with the J5 mutant of *E. coli* 0111:B4, which exhibit extensive serological cross-reactivity with a variety of Gram-negative bacteria [44-52]. Three laboratories have generated human monoclonal antibodies recognizing cross-reactive determinants on lipopolysaccharides [53-55]. In two of these studies, animal models were described.

Young et al. [56] described a murine IgM mab to *S. minnesota* that gave modest protection to live *E. coli* challenge. In other work [578] Young claimed that the antibody only gave protection when a serum-sensitive strain was used for challenge. No protection was seen when the encapsulated *E. coli* strain K13 was used. When he used his best monoclonal, a murine IgM anti-J5, 0.3-0.4 mg iv was required to protect mice against *E. coli* 085:H9 or two serotypes of *P. aeruginosa* in infection models combined with sub-optimal doses of antibiotics. One of these antibodies, the Xomen 5 antibody has completed clinical testing [58] and is awaiting FDA approval for use in a subset of patients with sepsis.

Three groups have published on anti-endotoxin human monoclonals [59-61]. These antibodies were IgMs generated by EBV transformation and fusion to mouse-human heteromyelomas. Zeigler et al. [62] described that a human IgM monoclonal antibody directed against lipid A determinants abrogated the *in vivo* effect of LPS in the rabbit dermal Shwartzman reaction and protected mice against lethal Gram-negative bacteria infection. Larrick et al. [63] described a series of human monoclonals that bound to various epitopes in the LPS core region. One of these antibodies could be produced under serum-free conditions at several hundred milligrams/liter. These antibodies are the leading human monoclonals in clinical trials. The antibody described by Zeigler et al. is one of the antibodies being tested by Centocor. These antibodies demonstrate wide cross-species bacterial binding but *in vivo* testing is equivocal. Large doses of antibody (2-10 mg/mouse) are required if the antibodies are administered *after* infection. Obviously in the clinical setting treatment will take place after infection. Evaluation of these monoclonals in clinical trials is awaited with much anticipation.

Two human clinical studies using J5 antisera prophylactically have been reported. In the first of these [64], neutropenic patients received either one unit of preimmune serum or anti-J5 antiserum. No favorable effect was observed in this study. A second prophylactic trial tested the protective effect of J5 plasma given to intensive care unit patients at risk for Gram-negative infection [65, 66]. Shock was more common in the control group and mortality was higher.

The most recent J5 study [67] tested whether purified anti-J5 IgG was protective. A protective effect could not be demonstrated. A clinical trial of purified high titer anti-Re antibodies is in progress in Europe.

The generation of humabs recognizing type specific determinants on Gram-negative bacteria is a reasonable alternative to the J5 cross-reactive monoclonals. Type-specific horse antibodies recognizing typhoid and pneumococcus immunotypes were used from the turn of the century until the beginning of the antibiotic era in the 1940's. Although the diversity of possible immunotypes of Gram-negative bacteria is large, a subset of these are known to be responsible for most of the invasive bacteremias. Several groups are trying to generate a limited number of type-specific humabs and administer a cocktail of antibodies. A humab providing protection for *E. coli* K1 and *Neisseria meningitidis* group B infections has been described [68].

The cocktail approach is being tried for *Pseudomonas aeruginosa* [69-73]. In model systems, murine monoclonal antibodies recognizing a single immunotype were much more effective than those recognizing a core determinant that was shared between *Pseudomonas* species. If the cocktail approach is to prove effective, it may be necessary to add humabs that neutralize various virulence factors. In the case of *Pseudomonas* infections, humabs have also been generated to exotoxin A [74].

Humabs have been reported that recognize *Haemophilus influenzae* type B capsular polysaccharide [75]. The successful introduction of an *H. influenzae* type B capsular polysaccharide vaccine [76] has made the clinical use of these humabs less attractive than originally anticipated, however, a safe humab for this life-threatening disease may still be developed for pediatric use in conjunction with the vaccines.

Anti-*Mycobacterium leprae* humabs have been reported [77]. In view of the central role of cell-mediated immunity in resistance and recovery from this disease, these reagents are unlikely to find clinical application. Nevertheless, these antibodies and those made by patients suffering from other infectious diseases can be used to probe the human humoral immune response, to clone antigens recognized by the humabs, and to investigate antibody mediated autoimmunity initiated by micro-organisms.

6.4.2 Viral and Chlamydial Targets

Anti-viral humabs (see Tab. 6-4) are especially attractive therapeutic targets because organic anti-viral therapeutics have been difficult to develop. Primary cytomegalovirus (CMV) infection is a major problem in immunosuppressed patients, allograft recipients and premature infants and CMV immune globulin effectively reduces infection [78]. Several groups have generated CMV neutralizing humabs [79-81] and clinical trials are underway [82].

Tab. 6-4 Human monoclonal antibodies: Viral and chlamydial and parasitic targets.

Chlamydia [89]
Cytomegalovirus
Rabies [90]
Rubella [91]
Hepatitis A [92]
Hepatitis B [93-95]
X31 Influenza virus [96]
Herpes simplex virus [97]
Measles (SSPE) virus [98, 99]
Varicella zoster [100]
Epstein Barr Virus [101-103]
Human T cell leukemia virus [104]
Human immunodeficiency virus (HIV) [105, 106]
Malaria antigens

Humabs neutralizing hepatitis B virus will replace the antisera currently used after acute exposure to this agent. These humabs may also be useful for so-called active-passive immunization of at-risk infants. A very large population of infants particularly in less developed countries become chronically infected in the perinatal period. Evidence suggests that administration of immune sera in this setting will prevent lifelong infection and could have an impact on the prevalence of the most common human cancer in the world, hepatitis B positive hepatoma. The widespread use of anti-hepatitis A antisera suggests that the humabs generated to this target may also find clinical application.

A minor yet important target for which humabs will find a niche is for the treatment of varicella zoster infections. These humabs may have to be developed as orphan drugs (that is, drugs for rare diseases, the development of which is supported by the US governement) given the small numbers of patients.

The acquired immunodeficiency syndrome (AIDS) with its viral agents, human immunodeficiency viruses, is the major infectious viral disease problem on the immediate horizon. Many groups are generating humabs that recognize one or more strains of the HIVs. Many of these humabs recognize the parts of the envelop gene product gp160. At present, there is no evidence that a humoral immune response can prevent or change the pattern of HIV infection in people or animals with these devastating viral infections. The viruses are known to undergo rapid mutation (five times the rate of influenza). Perhaps more importantly they can spread by cell to cell contact and reside permanently out of reach of humoral immunity inside the mononuclear phagocytes scattered throughout the body. Trials are underway to test the efficacy of a high titer anti-HIV antiserum in the prevention of neonatal AIDS. The dismal failure of all vaccine attempts and of passive serum to delay the spread of the virus in subhuman primate models is very discouraging. It is possible that anti-viral humabs attached to toxins or engineered to bring cytotoxic cells into contact with infected cells might improve the potency of the antibody approach.

Several other viral and chlamydial humabs have been generated and are listed in Tab. 6-4. At the present time there is limited clinical interest in any of these for therapeutic purposes.

6.4.3 Parasitic Targets

The major therapeutic target of interest among parasitic diseases is malaria. Much less is known about the humoral immune response of humans suffering from other parasitic diseases. Passively administered humabs may have therapeutic potential in acute *Falciparum* malaria. IgM and IgG humabs have been generated by Schmidt-Ullrich et al. [83] and by Udomsangpetch et al. [84].

6.5 Antibody Inhibition of the Immunoinflammatory Cascade

Severe infections of all types initiate an immunoinflammatory cascade that is characterized by the activation of complement, blood clotting, cellular activation and adhesion to endothelial cells accompanied by the release of numerous mediators such as tumor necrosis factor, interleukin 1, gamma interferon, platelet activating factor etc. A review of this cascade and the points that can be inhibited by antibodies is published elsewhere [85].

6.6 Conclusions

There is enormous potential for the use of humabs in the treatment of various infectious diseases. In the near future humabs will replace most antisera. Low doses of type-specific monoclonals have consistently given protection against various Gram-negative bacteria or their endotoxins. Less convincing are results with the cross-reactive anti-LPS core monoclonals. A rational approach will use cocktails of human monoclonal antibodies of limited cross-reactivity covering the most common bacterial serotypes. To date there has been limited development of anti-viral drugs, therefore anti-viral neutralizing humabs will be very useful. Other potential uses of humabs for therapy of infectious diseases include anti-idiotype vaccines and mabs that modulate the immunoinflammatory cascade.

6.7 References

1. Kohler, G. and Milstein, C., *Nature* (1975), **256**, 495-497.
2. Mudgett-Hunter, M.,Anderson, W., Haber, E. and Margolies, M.N., *Mol. Immunol.* (1985), **22**, 477-488.
3. Shawler, D. L., Bartholomew, R. M., Smith, L. M. and Dillman, R. O., *J. Immunol.* (1985), **135**, 1530-1535.
4. Schroff, R., Foon, K., Beatty, S., Oldham, R. and Morgan, A., Jr., *Cancer Res.* (1985), **45**, 879-885.
5. McCabe, R. P., Peters, L. C., Haspel, M. V., et al., *Cancer Res.* (1989), **48**, 4348-4353.
6. Nose, M. and Wigzell, H., *Proc. Natl. Acad. Sci. U.S.A.* (1983), **80**, 6632-6636.
7. Borrebaeck, C. A. K., Danielsson, L. and Moller, S. A., *Science* (1988), **85**, 3995-3999.
8. McCune, J. M., Namikawa, R., Kaneshima, H., et al., *Science* (1988), **241**, 1632-1639.
9. Larrick, J. W. and Bourla, J. M., *J. Biol. Response Mod.* (1986), **5**, 379-393.
10. Thompson, K. M., *Immunol. Today* (1988), **9**, 113-117.
11. James, K. and Bell, G. T., *J. Immunol. Meth.* (1987), **100**, 5-40.
12. Morrison, S. L., Johnson, M. J., Herzenberg, L. A. and Oi, V. T., *Proc. Natl. Acad. Sci. U.S.A.* (1984), **81**, 6851-6855.
13. Boulianne, G. L., Hozumi, N. and Shulman, M. J., *Nature* (1984), **312**, 644-646.
14. Morrison, S. L., and Oi, V. T., *Adv. Immunol.* (1989), **44**, 65-92.
15. Steplewski, Z., Sun, L. K., Shearman, C. W. et al., *Proc. Natl. Acad. Sci. U.S.A.* (1988), **85**, 4852-4856.
16. Bruggemann, M., Williams, G. T., Bindo, C. I., et al., *J. Exp. Med.* (1987), **166**, 1351-1361.
17. Jones, P. T., Dear, P. H., Foote, J., et al., *Nature* (1986), **321**, 522-525.
18. Verhoeyen, M., Milstein, C. and Winter, G., *Science* (1988), **239**, 1534-1536.
19. Riechmann, L., Clark, M., Waldmann, H. and Winter, G., *Nature* (1988), **332**, 323-327.
20. Waldmann, H., Hale, G., Clark, M., et al., *Prog. Allergy* (1988), **45**, 16-30.
21. Hale, G., Dyer, M. J. S., Clark, M. R. et al., *Lancet* (1988), **ii**, 1394-1399.
22. Larrick, J. W., Danielsson, L., Brenner, C. A., Abrahamson, M., Fry, K. E. and Borrebaeck, C., *Biochem. Biophys. Res. Comm.* (1989), **160**, 1250-1256.
23. Larrick, J. W., Danielsson, L., Brenner, C. A., Wallace, E., Abrahamson, M., Fry, K. E. and Borrebaeck, C., *Biotechnology* (1989), **7**, 934-939.
24. Chiang, Y. L., Dong, R. and Larrick, J. W., *Biotechniques* (1989), **7**, 360-366.
25. Khazaeli, M. B., Saleh, M. N., Wheeler, R. H., et al., *J. Natl. Cancer Inst.* (1988), **80**, 937-942.
26. Steihm, E. R., et al., *Ann. Intern. Med.* (1987), **107**, 367-382.

27. Kozbor, D., Roder, J., Chang, T., Steplewski, Z. and Koprowski, H., *Hybridoma* (1982), **1**, 323-328.
28. Larrick, J., Truitt, K., Raubitschek, A., Senyk, G. and Wang, J., *Proc. Natl. Acad. Sci. U.S.A.* (1983), **80**, 6376-6380.
29. Chiorazzi, N., Wasserman, R. and Kunkel, H., *J. Exp. Med.* (1982), **156**, 930-935.
30. Gigliotti, F. and Insel, R., *J. Clin. Invest.* (1982), **70**, 1306-1309.
31. Olsson, L., Mazauric, T., Vincent-Falquet, J. and Armand, J., *Dev. Biol. Stand.* (1984), **57**, 87-91.
32. Tsuchiya, S., Yokoyama, S., Yoshie, O. and Ono, Y., *J. Immunol.* (1980), **124**, 1970-1976.
33. Brade, H. and Galanos, C., *Infect. Immun.* (1983), **42**, 250-256.
34. Tate, W. J., III., Douglas, H. and Braude, A. I., *Ann. N.Y. Acad. Sci.* (1966), **133**, 746-762.
35. Chedid, L., Parant, M., Parant, F. and Boyer, F., *J. Immunol.* (1968), **292-301.**
36. Braude, A. I., Ziegler, E. J., Douglas, H. and McClutchan, J. A., *J. Infect. Dis.* (1977), **136**, S167-S173.
37. Johns, M. A., Bruins, S. C. and McCabe, W. R., *Infect. Immun.* (1977), **17**, 9-15.
38. Ziegler, E. J., McCutchan, J. A., Fierer, J., et al., *N. Engl. J. Med.* (1983), **37**, 1225-1230.
39. Baumgartner, J. D., Glauser, M. P., McCutchan, J. A., et al., *Lancet* (1985), **ii**, 59-63.
40. Calandra, T., Schellekens, J., Verhoef, J., et al., 4th International Symposium on Infections in the Immunocompromised Host, Ronneby Brunn, Sweden, (1986), **Abstr. N. 128**.
41. Greisman, S. E. and Johnston, C. A., *J. Infect. Dis.* (1988), **157**, 54-64.
42. Gigliotti, F. and Shenep, J. L., *J. Infect. Dis.* (1985), **151**, 1005-1011.
43. Ziegler, E., McCutchan, J., Fierer, J., et al., *N. Engl. J. Med.* (1982), **307**, 1225-1230.
44. Miner, K. M., Manyak, C. L., Williams, E. J., et al., *Infect. Immun.* (1986), **52**, 56-62.
45. Dunn, D. L., Ewald, D. C., Chandan, N. and Cerra, F. B., *Arch. Surg.* (1986), **121**, 58-62.
46. Mutharia, L. M., Crockford, G., Bogard, W. C., Jr. and Hancock, R. E. W., *Infect. Immun.* (1984), **45**, 631-636.
47. Nelles, M. J. and Niswander, C. A., *Infect. Immun.* (1984), **46**, 677-681.
48. Mehta, N. D., Thesis, University of London, (1987).
49. Appelmelk, B. J., Verweij-van Vught, J. J., Maaskant, J. J., et al., *Antonie van Leeuwenhoek* (1986), **52**, 537-542.
50. Appelmelk, B. J., Verweij-van Vught, J. J., Maaskant, J. J., et al., *F.E..S. Microbiol. Lett.* (1987), **40**, 71-74.
51. Coughlin, R. T., Zissimos, E. M., Kligarraff, C., et al., *J. Immunol. Immunopharmacol.* (1986), **6 (suppl.)**, 260-270.
52. Dunn, D. L., Bogard, W. C., Jr., and Cerra, F. B., *Surgery* (1985), **98**, 283-289.
53. Teng, N. H., Kaplan, H. S., Hebert, J., et al., *Proc. Natl. Acad. Sci. U.S.A.* (1985), **82**, 1790-1794.
54. Bogard, W. C., Jr., Hornberger, E. and Kung, P., *In:* Engleman, E. G., Foung, S. K. H., Larrick, J. and Raubitchek, A. (eds.) Human hybridomas and monoclonal antibodies. Plenum Press, New York, (1985), 95-112.
55. Pollack, M., Raubitschek, A. A. and Larrick, J. W., *J. Clin. Invest.* (1987), **79**, 1421-1427.
56. Young, L. S., Alam, S. and Gascon, R., *Clin. Res.* (1982), **30**, 552A.
57. Young, L. S., *Infection* (1982), **12**, 303-307.
58. Harkonen, S., Scannon, P., Mischak, R. P., et al., *Antimicrob. Agents. Chemother.* (1988), **32**, 710-716.
59. Bogard, W., Hornberger, E. and Kung, P., *In:* Englemann, E., Foung, S., Larrick, J. and Raubitschek, A. (eds.) Human hybridomas and monoclonal antibodies. Plenum Press, New York, (1985), 905-112.
60. Teng, N., Kaplan, H., Hebert, J., et al., *Proc. Natl. Acad. Sci. U.S.A.* (1985), **82**, 179-184.
61. Larrick, J., Jahnsen, M., Senyk, G., Weiss, S. and Watson, K., *In:* Friedman, H. (ed.) The Immunology and Immunopharmacology of Bacterial Endotoxins. Plenum Press, New York, (1986), 75-81.
62. Zeigler, E. J. and Teng, N. N. H., *J. Immunol. Immunopharmacol.* (1986), **6 (suppl.)**, 139-141.
63. Larrick, J.W., Jahnsen, M., Senyk, G., Weiss, S. and Watson, K., *In:* Friedman, H. (ed.) The Immunobiology and Immunopharmacology of Bacterial Endotoxins. Plenum Press, New York, (1986), 75-81.
64. McCutchan, J. A., Wolf, J. L., Zeigler, E. J. and Braude, A. I., *Schweiz. Med. Wschr.* (1987), **113 (suppl. 14)**, 40-45.
65. Calandra, T., Glauser, M. P., Schellekens, J., et al., *J. Infect. Dis.* (1988), **158**, 312-319.
66. Baumgartner, J., Glauser, M., McCuchan, J., Zeigler, E., et al., *Lancet* (1985), **ii**, 59-65.

67. Baumgartner, J. D. and Glauser, M. P., *Rev. Infect. Dis.* (1987), **9**, 194-205.
68. Raff, H. V., Devereux, D., Shufort, W., et al., *J. Infect. Dis.* (1988), **157**, 118-126.
69. Larrick, J., Hart, S., Lippman, D., Glembourtt, M., et al., *In:* Strelkelkaus, A. (ed.) Human hybridomas: diagnostic and therapeutic applications. Marcel-Dekker, New York, (1986), 65-80.
70. Lang, A. B., Furer, E., Senyk, G., Larrick, J. W. and Cryz, S. J., Jr., *Infect. Immun.* (1989), in press.
71. Lang, A. B., Furer, E., Larrick, J. W. and Cryz, S. J., Jr., *J. Immunol.* (1989), submitted.
72. Zweerink, H. J., Gammon, M. C., Hutchison, C. F., et al., *Infect. Immun.* (1988), **56**, 1873-1879.
73. Lam, J. S., MacDonald, L. A. and Lam, M. Y., *Infect. Immun.* (1987), **55**, 2854-2856.
74. Larrick, J., Dyer, B. and Senyk, G., *In:* Engleman, E., Foung, S., Larrick, J., Raubitschek, A. (eds.) Human hybridomas and monoclonal antibodies. Plenum Press, New York, (1985), 49-65.
75. Hunter, K., Jr., Fischer, G., Hemming, V., Wilson, S., Hartzman, R. and Woody, J., *Lancet* (1982), **ii**, 798-799.
76. Peltola, H., Kayhty, H., Virtanen, M. and Makela, P., *N. Engl. J. Med.* (1984), **310**, 1561-1565.
77. Atlaw, T., Kozbor, D. and Roder, J., *Infect. Immun.* (1985), **49**, 104-110.
78. Meyers, J. D., Leszyzczynski, J., Zaia, J. A., Flournoy, N., Newton, B., Syndman, D. R., Wright, G. G., Levin, M. J. and Thomas, E. D., *Ann. Int. Med.* (1983), **98**, 442-446.
79. Emanuel, D., Gold, J., Colacino, J., Lopez, C. and Hammerling, U., *J. Immunol.* (1984), **133**, 2202-2205.
80. Amadei, C., Michelson, S., Frot, J., Fruchart, M., et al., *Dev. Biol. Stand* (1984), **57**, 283-286.
81. Foung, S. K. H., Perkins, S., Bradshaw, P., Rowe, J., Rabin, L. B., Reyes, G. R. and Lennette, E. T., *J. Infect. Dis.* (1989), **159**, 436-443.
82. Ehrlich, P. H., Moustafa, Z. A., Justice, J. C., et al., *Clin. Chem.* (1988), **34**, 1681-1688.
83. Schmidt-Ullrich, R., Brown, J., Whittle, R. and Lin, P., *J. Exp. Med.* (1986), **163**, 179-189.
84. Udomsangpetch, R., Lundgren, K., Berzins, et al., *Science* (1986), **231**, 55-59.
85. Larrick, J. W., *J. Critical Care* (1989), in press.
86. Brodeur, B., Lagace, L., Larose, Y., Martin, M., et al., *In:* Schook, B. (ed.) Monoclonal Antibodies. Marcel Dekker, New York, (1986), 51-59.
87. Steinitz, M., Tamir, S. and Goldfarb, A., *J. Immunol.* (1984), **132**, 877-882.
88. Schwaber, J., Posner, M., Schlossman, S. and Lazarus, H., *Hum. Immunol.* (1984), **9**, 137-142.
89. Rosen, A., Persson, K. and Klein, G., *J. Immunol.* (1983), **130**, 2899-2899.
90. Hilfenhaus, J., Kanzy, E., Kohler, R. and Willems, W., *Behring Inst. Mitt.* (1986), **80**, 31-40.
91. van Meel, F., Steenbakkers, P. and Oomen, J., *J. Immunol. Meth.* (1985), **80**, 267-280.
92. Beasley, R., Hwang, L., Leu, C., et al., *Lancet* (1981), **ii**, 388-393.
93. Burnett, K., Leung, J. and Marinis, J., *In:* Engleman, E., Foung, S., Larrick, J. and Raubitschek, A. (eds.) Human hybridomas and monoclonal antibodies. Plenum Press, New York, (1985), 113-133.
94. Ichimori, Y., Sasano, K., Itoh, H., Hitosumachi, S., et al., *Biochem. Biophys. Res. Commun.* (1985), **129**, 26-38.
95. Stricker, E., Tiebout, R., Lelie, P. and Zeijlemaker, W., *Scand. J. Immunol.* (1985), **22**, 337-345.
96. Crawford, D., Callard, R., Muggeridge, M., Mitchell, D., Zanders, E. and Beverley, P., *J. Gen. Virol.* (1983), **64**, 697-700.
97. Seigneurin, J., Desgranges, C., Siegneurin, D., et al., *Science* (1983), **221**, 173-175.
98. Masuho, Y., Sugano, T., Matsumoto, Y., Sawada, S. and Tomibe, K., *Biochem. Biophys. Res. Commun.* (1986), **135**, 495-505.
99. Evans, L., Maragos, C. and May, J., *Immunol. Lett.* (1984), **8**, 39-50.
100. Croce, C., Linnenbach, A., Hall, W., Steplewski, Z. and Koprowski, H., *Nature* (1980), **288**, 488-489.w
101. Foung, S., Perkins, S., Koropchak, C., et al., *J. Infect. Dis.* (1985), **52**, 280-285.
102. Ritts, R., Jr., Ruiz-Arguelles, A. and Weyl, K., *Int. J. Cancer* (1983), **31**, 133-151.
103. Koizumi, S., Fujiwara, S., Kikuta, H., et al., *Virology* (1986), **150**, 161-170.
104. Matsushita, S., Robert-Gurhoff, M., Trepel, J., Cossman, J., Mitsuya, H. and Broder, S., *Proc. Natl. Acad. Sci. U.S.A.* (1986), **83**, 2672-2677.
105. Evans, L., Homsy, J., Morrow, W., Gaston, I., et al., *J. Immunol.* (1988), **140**, 941-943.
106. Banapour, B., Rosenthal, K., Rabin, L., Sharma, V., et al., *J. Immunol.* (1987), **138**, 4027-4033.

Index